# Textbook of Agada Tantra evam Vidhi Vaidyaka

**Dr. Kausambi D. Vaghela**

**Dr. Rutviksinh D. Jadeja**

KORYFI GROUP
of Media & Publications

# Textbook of Agada Tantra evam Vidhi Vaidyaka

**Author:**
**Dr. Kausambi D. Vaghela**
**Dr. Rutviksinh D. Jadeja**

**ISBN: 9789347166297**

**Price: Rs. 999/-**

First Published in December, 2025

***Publisher & Printer:***
**Koryfi Group of Media and Publications**
**Address:** B-515, 5th Floor, Shalin Square, Nr. Lalgebi Circle,
S. P. Ring Road, Hathijan, Ahmedabad, Gujarat, India - 382445
**Phone:** +91-635 635 60 70 | **Email:** editor@koryfigroup.org
**Website:** book.koryfigroup.org

***Cover Designer:***
Harsh Koshti

# Foreword

It gives me great honor to write the foreword for this valuable work, A Textbook of Agada tantra. This book is a significant contribution to the field of Ayurveda, offering a well-balanced blend of scholarly knowledge and practical insights into the subject.

Dr. Kausambi D. Vaghela, the author, brings with her vast experience and a deep-rooted passion for Agada tantra. Her clear explanations and well-researched content not only educate but also inspire readers. The book reflects her commitment to knowledge dissemination and her sincere effort to make a lasting impact on students and practitioners alike.

What makes this book truly commendable is its timeless relevance. It will undoubtedly serve as an essential resource for second-year Ayurveda students, while also enriching the understanding of anyone who delves into its pages.

I sincerely applaud Dr. Kausambi D. Vaghela for this remarkable contribution and encourage every reader to approach this text with enthusiasm and an inquisitive mind.

**Prof. Dr. D. B. Vaghela**
**M.D. (Shalakya), Ph.D. (Ayu)**
**HOD Shalakya Tantra**
**ITRA, Jamnagar.**

# Foreword

In an era where clarity and precision are as valued as depth of knowledge, Concised Textbook of Agada Tantra by Dr. Kausambi D. Vaghela arrives as a refreshing and much-needed contribution to Ayurvedic literature.

Agada Tantra, the branch of Ayurveda that deals with toxicology, is both ancient and profound – steeped in tradition, yet vital to modern practice. What Dr. Kausambi achieves in this volume is no small feat: the distillation of centuries of wisdom into a compact, accessible, and intellectually stimulating form. This is not just a textbook; it is a guide, a companion, and an invitation to explore one of the most dynamic disciplines in Ayurveda.

With thoughtful organization, lucid language, and a learner-focused approach, the author has transformed what is often considered a challenging subject into a readable and relevant narrative. Whether you are a student navigating your second year of BAMS, a teacher seeking teaching clarity, or a lifelong learner of Ayurveda, this book offers both substance and simplicity.

In these pages, ancient insights meet modern minds. It is a commendable step toward making Ayurvedic toxicology not only understandable but also applicable in today's context.

I congratulate Dr. Kausambi Vaghela for her dedication and scholarly excellence, and I am confident that this textbook will become a valued asset on the desks – and in the minds – of many Ayurvedic scholars to come.

Let this concise journey through Agada Tantra begin.

**Dr. Shraddha Joshi**
**M.S. (Shalakya), Ph.D. (Ayu)**
**Medical Officer, Govt. of Uttarakhand.**

# Preface

It gives me immense pleasure to write the preface for this valuable work authored by Dr. Kausambi D. Vaghela. The book, The Textbook of Agada tantra is a thoughtful and well-researched contribution to the field of Ayurveda. The author has presented the subject matter with remarkable clarity, depth, and precision, making it accessible to both students and professionals alike.

In this era of rapidly evolving knowledge, such comprehensive efforts are essential for guiding readers toward a balanced understanding of traditional wisdom and modern perspectives. The systematic arrangement of chapters, lucid explanations, and practical examples reflect the author's dedication and scholarly insight.

I am confident that this book will serve as a reliable companion for learners, teachers, and researchers, enriching their understanding and inspiring further exploration.

I extend my heartfelt congratulations to Dr. Kausambi D. Vaghela for this commendable work and wish the book every success.

**Dr. Rutviksinh D. Jadeja**
**3rd Year Resident,**
**Department of Anaesthesiology,**
**B. J. Medical College, Ahmedabad.**

# Acknowledgments

It is with great pleasure that I express my sincere gratitude to all those who have contributed, directly or indirectly, to the successful completion of this book, The Textbook of Agadtantra, authored by Dr. Kausambi D. Vaghela. The author is thankful to the authors whose reference have been used in this book.

The author is immensely thankful to her father- Dr. D. B. Vaghela, mother- Mrs. Maheshwariba D. Vaghela and husband- Dr. Rutviksinh D. Jadeja.

Finally, our deepest thanks go to the readers, for whom this book has been written. It is our hope that this work will serve as a meaningful contribution to the field and a useful reference for students, teachers.

**Dr. Raj H. Dethaliya**
**3rd Year Resident,**
**Department of Anaesthesiology,**
**B. J. Medical College, Ahmedabad.**

# Table of Content

# Ch. 1
# Concepts of Agada-Tantra [Clinical Toxicology]

## 1.1 Agada-Tantra and Clinical Toxicology:

- **Nirukti:**
    - Agada + Tantra = Agada -Tantra
    - Agada is the antidote of Gada (poison).
    - Tantra is a science.

- **Definition:**

    अगदतन्त्रंनामसर्पकीटलूतामूषीकादिदष्टविषव्यञ्जनार्थंविविधविषसं योगोपशमनार्थंच ।। (सु.सू.१/१४)

Agada-Tantra is intended for diagnosis, signs symptoms and management of various poisonings such as bites of Sarpa (snake), Kita (insects), Luta (spiders), Mushaka (rats), etc.

- **Clinical Toxicology:**

The discipline which deals with avoiding of adverse effects of drugs and radiation and its management. It also does research on various drugs to avoid drug related insults on human body.

## 1.2 Scope of Agada-Tantra:

- Protection of healthy individuals from poisons.
- Management of individuals afflicted with poisons.
- Most probably all the modern day diseases are caused as a result of pollution, intake of Viruddha ahara and non-intentional ingestion of metallic poisons from various unavoidable sources.
- As the industries grow, automobiles increase, there occurs a high amount of pollution resulting in diseases like cancer,

skin diseases and allergies.

- Incidence of these diseases increases with the passing time. These diseases may be produced due to acute or chronic exposure.
- Also the poisons when chronic, mostly are low potency and doesn't cause instant death but give fatal symptoms as remains in the body for a long time.
- Some substances act due to mutual contraindications where as some by improper purification and ingestion. Thus Agada-Tantra deals with all these causes, signs symptoms and its treatment and gives a thorough base for less exposure on long term.

## 1.3 Definition of Visha & poison, Synonyms, Visha Guna, Difference between Visha, Madya & Oja Guna, Visha Gati, Classification of Visha & poison, Sthavara & Jangama Visha Adhishthana.

विष् + कः The substance which pervades throughout the body speedily after consumption is Visha. That which causes Vishada (fear / grief / distress) is known as Visha.

- **Paribhasha:**

विषादजननत्वाच्च विष्मित्यभिधीयते। ( सु .क. ३/२१)

Visha is the substance which when consumed in an impure form or in an improper (mostly high) quantity than induces fatal symptoms either causing death or ill health. Such a substance is called as Visha.

- **Definition of poison:**

The substance which on ingestion, inhaling or even just on touch causes devil effects on body and proves to be fatal is poison.

- Synonyms of poison: Kshveda, Garala, Jivitapaham, Rasa, Mustaka, Gara.

- **Visha Guna: - 10**

  लघु रूक्षमाशु विशदं व्यवायि तीक्ष्णं विकासि सूक्ष्मं च ।
  उष्णमनिर्देश्यरसं दशगुणमुक्तं विषं तज्ज्ञेः। (च. चि. २३/२४)

**Visha Guna Visha Karma:**

1. Laghu: Duchikitsya (difficult to treat)
2. Ruksha: Vata prakopaka
3. Ashu / Ashukari (quick acting & destructive): Destroys the tissues quickly
4. Vishada: Does not adhere to any place
5. Vyavayi (pervading) Spreads within the whole body quickly; before undergoing digestion
6. Tikshna Causes Moha (delusion) and breaks Marma-bhanda (support of vital organs)
7. Vikasi (slackening) Slows & destroys functioning of Dosha, Dhatu & Mala
8. Sukshma Enters into all the organs at the minute level and causes abnormalities
9. Ushna Pitta & Rakta prakopaka
10. Anirdesha / Avyakta Rasa(indistinct taste) / Avipaki (indigestible): Not perceivable due to indistinctive taste / Difficult to expel due to indigestibility.

- **Difference between Visha, Madya, Oja:**

**1. Visha:** लघु रूक्षमाशु विशदं व्यवायि तीक्ष्णं विकासि सूक्ष्म च।
उष्णमनिर्देश्यरसं दशगुणमुक्तं विषं तद्ग्नेयं।। (च.चि.२३/२४)

**2. Oja:** गुरु शीतं मृदु श्लक्ष्णं बहलं मधुरं स्थिरं।
प्रसन्नं पिच्छिलं स्निग्धमोजो दशगुणं स्मृतं।। (च.चि.२४/३१)

**3. Madya:** लघूष्णतीक्ष्ण सूक्ष्माम्लव्यवय्याशुगमेव च।
रुक्षं विकाशि विशदं मद्यंदशगुणं स्मृतम।। (च. चि. २४/३०)

Table 1.1 Difference between Visha, Madya, Oja

| Visha | Madya | Oja |
|---|---|---|
| Laghu | Laghu | Guru |
| Ruksha | Ruksha | Snigdha |
| Tikshna | Tikshna | Mrudu |
| Ushna | Ushna | Sheeta |
| Sukshma | Sukshma | Bahula |
| Ashukari | Ashukari | Prasada |
| Vyavayi | Vyavayi | Sthira |
| Vikasi | Vikasi | Slaksna |
| Vishada | Vishada | Pichhila |
| Anirdeshya Rasa | Amla | Madhura |

- **Visha Gati:**

जङ्गमं स्यादधोभागमूर्ध्वभागं तु मूलजम्।
तस्माद्दंष्ट्राविषम मौलं हन्ति मौलं च दंष्ट्रजम्।।१७।।
(च. चि. २३/१७)

Jangama Visha moves downwards whereas Sthavara Visha moves upwards in the alimentary canal. Therefore, Jangama Visha cures poisoning of Sthavara Visha, and vice-versa

- **Classification of Visha and poison:**

Table 1.2 Classification of Visha

| Acharya Charak and Acharya Sushruta | Ashtanga Hridaya | Bhavprakasha | Rasatarangini |
|---|---|---|---|
| • Sthavara, Jangama | • Akritrim: Sthavara, Jangama | • Akritrim: Sthavara, Jangama | • Sthavara visha: Mahavisha, Upavisha |
| • Gara, Kritrim | • Kritrim: Gara visha | • Kritrim: Dushivisha, Garavisha | • Jangama visha |

Table 1.3 Classification of Poison

| 1. Corrosive poison | 2. Irritant poison | 3. Systemic poison |
|---|---|---|
| • Mineral acid: Hydrochloric acid, sulphuric acid | • Inorganic: Metallic and non-metallic | • Cerebral: Opium, Dhatura, alcohol, ether |
| • Organic acid: Carbolic acid, acetic acid | • Vegetable: Castor oil, croton seeds | • Spinal poison |
| • Strong alkalies | • Animal: Snake bites, insect bites | • Cardiac poison.<br>• Asphaxiant poison |

- **Visha Adhishthana:**

*Sthavara visha:*

मूलं पत्रं फलं पुष्प त्वक क्षीर सार ऐव च।
निर्यासो धातवश्चैव कन्दश्च दशम स्मृतः।। (सु.क.३/३)

Roots, leaves, fruits, flowers, bark, sap milk, pith, gum, minerals, bulb are the sites for poison in vegetation.

*Jangama visha:*

जंगमस्य विषस्य अधिष्ठान षोडश।
समासेन मया यानि विस्तरस्तेषु वक्ष्यते।।
तत्र दृष्टनिश्वासःदंष्ट्रा नखमूत्र पुरिषलार्तव।
मुखसंदंश विधिर्तुण्डा पित्तशुकशवानिति।। (सु.क.३/३–४)

Site, breath, teeth, nails, urine, stool, semen, saliva, menstrual blood, stings, belching, anus, bones, bile, bristles and dead body of animals.

## 1.4 Difference between Poison, Venom, Toxin:

Table 1.4 Difference between Poison, Venom, Toxin

| Poison | Venom | Toxin |
|---|---|---|
| Can be produced by plants and animals. | Produced by animals. | Produced by organisms which can potentially cause harm. |
| It can enter in body by ingestion, inhalation | It is delivered from a bite or insect sting. | Low levels can cause major diseases. |
| It can also start effect by a touch on skin. | It is present in venom glands of animals and secreted by teeth, fangs. | Requires specific sensitive analytical instruments for its detection. |
| A protection mechanism from potential predator. | It is the mechanism to kill the predator or a prey. | When treatment started early, the potential harm can be reduced. |
| It is a non-aggressive attack by the animal. | It is an aggressive defence mechanism. | May include even some medicines which are useful in small doses but harmful in large dose. |
| Delivered to the prey non -actively. | It is actively delivered to the prey. | It is usually a single molecule. |
| Lethal if absorbed in large quantities. | Lethal even on exposure to small quantity. | They are identified based on their delivery route. |
| Eg: Mushrooms, fishes. | Eg: Cobra, scorpions. | Eg: Bacillus anthracis, Botulinum toxin. |

## 1.5 Routes of Poison Administration:

- **Local routes:** Skin, Eyes, Nose, Vagina, Rectum, Urethra.

- **Systemic routes:**

1. Oral: Painless, cheap and most convenient.
2. Sublingual: The fastest route of administration.
3. Inhalation, Rectal.
4. Parenteral: IM, IV, Intradermal, Subcutaneous.

## 1.6 Mode of action of Visha and poison:

Table 1.5 Mode of action of Visha and poison

| गुण | पंचभौतिक संगठन | गुणकर्म | कर्म |
|---|---|---|---|
| लघु | अग्नि, वायु, आकाश | कफवृद्धिकर, वातघ्न | लंघन |
| रूक्ष | अग्नि, वायु, पृथ्वि | वातवृद्धिकर, कफघ्न | शोषण |
| उष्ण | अग्नि | पित्तवृद्धिकर, वातघ्न | स्वेदन |
| तीक्ष्ण | अग्नि | पित्तवृद्धिकर, कफघ्न | शोधन |
| सूक्ष्म | अग्नि, वायु, आकाश | वातवृद्धिकर | विवरण |
| विशद | Except जल | वातवृद्धिकर | क्षालन |

- **Mode of action of poison:**

Toxic kinetics: The process of absorption, distribution, biotransformation and excretion of chemicals.

Image 1.1 Steps of toxicokinetics

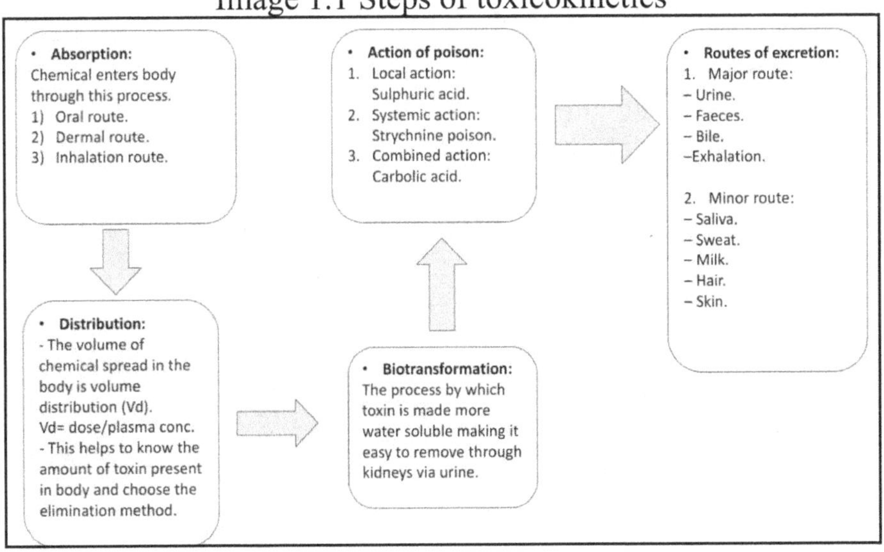

## 1.7 Factors modifying action of poison:

- **Age:** Children and elders more affected.
- **Dose:** Larger the dose, worse the effects causing intense and rapid poisoning.
- **Allergens:** Person allergic to substance when comes in its contact may cause severe and immediate effects even if minute dosage.
- **Area:** Larger the area, severe the effect.
- **State of poison:** Volatile substance acts fast and produces severe effects.
- **Route:** Parenteral route acts faster than the oral route.
- **Tolerance:** Females < Males, Sick < Healthy.

## 1.8 Visha Vardhaka Bhava and Visha Sankata:

- **Visha Vardhaka Bhava:**(अ.हृ.उ. ३५/६१–६३)

क्षुधातृष्णाघर्मदौर्बल्यक्रोधशोकभयश्रमैः ।
अजीर्णवर्चोद्रवतापित्तमारुतवृद्धिभि : ।।
तिलपुष्पफलाघ्राणभूबाष्पघनगर्जितैः ।
हस्तिमूषिकवादिन्नत्रनि स्वनैविषसंकटैः ।।
पुरोवातोत्पलामोदनदनैवर्धते ।।

Hunger, thirst, heat, weakness, anger, grief, exhaustion, indigestion, diarrhea, smelling flowers of Tila, thunders, sounds of elephant, mice and exposure to cold winds.

- **Visha Sankat:**(अ.हृ.उ.४०)

Prakruti: पित्त प्रकृति
Kala: वर्षा ऋतु, ग्रीष्म ऋतु
Anna: कटु तिक्त रस
Dosha: पित्तदोष
Dushya: रक्त

## 1.9 Visha Vega:

धात्वंतरेषु याः सप्त कलाः सम्परिकीर्तिता।
तास्वेकैकां अतिक्रम्य वेगं प्रकुरुते विशं। (सु . क. ४/४०)

Visha crossing over each of the seven Kalas (limitating membranes) successively situated in the midway region between two Dhatus, produces different phases of effect. This is termed as Visha Vega (velocity of poison).

**Number of Vegas:**

Acharya Charaka and Acharya Sushruta:
Human Beings 8
Animals 4
Birds 3

Acharya Sushruta has mentioned only 7 Vegas for Humans. There are seven Kalas in the body, and these Vegas (stages) appear when the Visha crosses the Kalas successively. After Saptama Vega, the Visha which spread by bite, returns back to Damshadesha (site of bite), and the Visha consumed orally returns to the Hridaya (heart) to cause death of the patient as the final stage. Thus, there is no contradiction between number of Vega of Acharya Charaka & Acharya Sushruta.

- **Visha Vega Lakshana:**

## 1. According to Acharya Charak:

Table 1.6 Visha vega according to Acharya Charak

| Vega sankhya | Vega lakshana | Meaning | Treatment |
|---|---|---|---|
| Prathama vega | तृणमोह्दंतहर्ष पृसेक्वमथुक्लमा भवत्यध्य वेग रस प्दोंश। (च. चि. 23) | Thirst, Moha, Tingling sensation in the teeth, Salivation, Chardi, Klama. | Agada yoga with Madhu & Ghrita. |
| Dwitiya vega | अश्रु प्रदोंशादीत्तीय तु ।। वैवर्णय भ्रम वेपथु मूर्छा जृम्भंग चिमिचिमतका: दुश्टपिशिता। (च. चि. 23) | Vaivarnya, Bhrama, Murccha, Jrimbha, Anga cimicima (tingling sensation in the limbs), Tamaka (dyspnea). | Virechana, Hridaya avacharana. |
| Tritiya vega | तृतीये मंडल कन्दुश्र्वयथुकोठा:। (च. चि. 23) | Mandala (circular eruptions), Kandu, Shvayathu (oedema), Kotha (urticaria). | Ksharagada with Madhu & Ambu, Agada Dravya, Nasya, Anjana. |
| Chaturtha vega | वातादि जाश्रचतुर्थे दाहछर्द्य अन्गशुल मुर्छ्ध्या:। (च. चि. 23) | Daha (burning), Chardi (vomiting), Angashula (bodyache), Murccha (unconsciousness). | Gomayarasa with Kapittha rasa, Madhu & Ghrita, Agada with Sneha. |
| Panchama vega | नीलदीनां तमश्र्च दर्शनं पंचमे वेग। (च. चि. 23) | Nila Darshana or Tamasa Darshana: observes everything as blue. | Ashchotana, Anjana, Nasya with Kakanda and Shirisha rasa, Agada with Madhuka kvatha & Madhu. |
| Sashtha vega | षष्ठे हिक्का:। (च. चि. 23) | Hiccups. | Atisara chikitsa. |
| Saptama vega | भंग: स्कंधस्य तु सप्तमे। (च. चि. 23) | Skandha bhanga (dislocation of shoulder girdle). | Use of Jangama Visha in case of Sthavara Visha, Avapidana Nasya. |
| Ashtama vega | अष्ठमे मरणं । (च. चि. 23) | Marana (death). | Palasha beeja with Shikhi-Pitta. |

### 2. According to Acharya Sushruta:

Table 1.7 Visha vega according Acharya Sushruta

| Vega sankhya | Kala | Symptoms | Treatment |
|---|---|---|---|
| Prathama vega | Rasa, Rakta. | Bluish tongue, fainting, dyspnoea. | Vamana, Agadapana |
| Dwitiya vega | Rakta, Mamsa. | Burning, pain in throat | Vamana, Virechana |
| Tritiya vega | Mamsa, Meda | Green eyes, hiccups, cough | Nasya, Anjana |
| Chaturtha vega | Meda, Kapha | Intestinal gurgling, heaviness in head | Sneha with Agadapana |
| Panchama vega | Kapha, Purisha | Pain in joints, large intestine | Madhu with Madhuka Kwatha |
| Sashtha vega | Purisha, Pitta | Diarrhoea, cutting pain in shoulders | Atisara Chikitsa, Nasya |
| Saptama vega | Pitta, Shukra. | Cessation of breathing | Awapeedaka Nasya |

Table 1.8 Visha Vega found in Animals

| Vega sankhya | Vega lakshana |
|---|---|
| Prathama Vega. | Depression, Bhrama. |
| Dwitiya Vega. | Vepana (trembling). |
| Tritiya Vega. | Shunya (feeling of emptiness), Manda-ahara Srasta-anga (sluggishness of the limbs), Marana (death). |
| Chaturtha vega. | Shvasa (Dyspnoea, Respiratory failure) Marana (death). |

### 3. Vishavega lakshana found in animals:

- **Visha Veganatara:**

येनान्तरेण तु कलां कलाकल्पं भिवनत्ति हि ।
समीर नो ह्यमानं तत्तू वेगान्तरं स्मृतम ।। (सु. क. ४/४१)

The interval which appears while poison is driven by Vayu from one Kala to another is known as Vega-antara (interval between phases).

### 1.10 Visha peeta lakshana: (अ.सं.उ. ४०/१२)

- **Visha peeta lakshana:**

चिम्चिमारं, कोठ, मण्डल, स्वेद, रोमहर्ष.

- **Visha peeta marana lakshana:**

नील औष्ठ, दन्त शैथिल्य, केशपतन, अंगभंग, विक्षेप, ना शिशिर लोमहर्ष, न अभिहते.

- **Visha Mukta Lakshana:**

प्रशान्त दोषं प्रकृतिस्थ धातु आहारकामं सममूत्र विटकं।
प्रसन्नवर्णेन्द्रिय चित्तचेष्ट वैद्यौ अवगच्चेद विषं मनंष्य।। (अ. सं.उ.४७/२७)

- प्रशान्त दोषः Normal Dosha Avastha.
- प्रकृतिस्थ धातुः Normalcy of Dhatus.
- आहारकामः Desire for food.
- सममूत्र विटकः Normal urine and stool.
- प्रसन्नवर्णेन्द्रियः Normalcy of compleÛion] sense organs and state of mind.
- चेष्टः Normalcy of activities.

- **Shanka-Visha:**

दुरन्ध्कारे विध्दस्य केनचिद् विष शंकया।
विषोद्वेगाज्ज्वरशछर्दिर्मूर्च्छा दहो अपी वा भवेत।।
ग्लानिर्मोहो अतिसारश्चाप्येतच्छ शंकाविष मतम्।।
(च – चि – २३ / २२१–२२२)

When a person is bitten by something (non-poisonous) in the pitch darkness, the fear or suspicion (Shanka) of being bitten by a poisonous creature causes manifestation of symptoms such as Jvara, Chardi, Murccha, Daha, Glani, Moha & Atisara .This condition is called Shanka-Visha.

For the treatment of this ailment, the wise physician should console the patient. He should be given Sharkara, Shuddha Gandhaka, Draksha, Payasya, Madhuka and Madhu along with Mantraputa Ambu (incanted water). The water should also be sprinkled.

**Multiple Choice Questions:**

1. Which of the following is not a synonym of अगदतन्त्र ?
A) कष्वेड B) गराल C) मुस्तक D) शास्त्र

2. According to चरक चकिति्सा स्थान, how many वषिगुण are mentioned?
A) 3 B) 5 C) 8 D) 10

3. Which among the following is not a factor for वषि संकट?
A) पकृति B) दुष्य C) दोष D) वकिृति

4. According to चरक चकिति्सा स्थान, which वषिवेग has a symptom हकि्का?
A) प्रथम B) चतुर्थ C) तृतीय D) षष्ठ

5. Which among the following is a वषिगुण?
A) गुरु B) तीक्ष्ण C) प्रसाद D) शीत

6. What is the गति of जंगम वषि?
A) उर्ध्व B) अधोC) तरि्यक D) उभय

7. Which is not a classification of वषि?
A) दूषी B) गर C) मद्य D) कृत्रमि

8. Which is not a step in Toxic kinetics?
A) Inhalation B) Distribution C) Absorption D) Excretion

9. Which is not a वषि वर्धक भाव?
A) क्षुधा B) तृष्णा C) आलस्य D) क्रोध

10. Which is a वषि मुक्त लक्षण?
A) दौर्बल्य B) प्रशांत दोष C) श्रम D) अजीर्ण

11. Which is not a वषिपीत लक्षण?
A) कोठ B) आहारकामं C) स्वेद D) मण्डल

12. येनान्तरण तु कलां कलाकल्पं भनि्वात्ती हि। is the shloka for ?
A) वषिवेग B) वषिवेगांतर C) वषिपीत D) वषिमुक्त

13. दुरन्ध्कलो वधि्दस्य केनचीत वशि शंकया। is the shloka for ?
A) वषिपीत B) वषिमुकत C) शंकावषि D) वषिवेग

14. लघु गुण of visha has which पंचभौतकि संगठन ?
A) वायु B) अगनि C) पृथवि D) अगनि + वायु + आकाश

15. Which of the following requires specific sensitive analytical instruments for its detection?
A) Poison B) Venom C) Toxin D) All of the above

**Answer Key for MCQs.**

| | |
|---|---|
| 1 | D |
| 2 | D |
| 3 | D |
| 4 | D |
| 5 | B |
| 6 | B |
| 7 | C |
| 8 | A |

| | |
|---|---|
| 9 | C |
| 10 | B |
| 11 | B |
| 12 | B |
| 13 | C |
| 14 | D |
| 15 | C |

# Ch. 2
# Visha Chikitsa
# [Management of Poisoning]

**2.1 Diagnosis of Poison in Living and Dead:**

The patient presenting with poison ingestion can be of type:

1. Acute poisoning.
2. Subacute poisoning.
3. Chronic poisoning.
4. Fulminant poisoning.

Diagnosis of poisoning is important, not only from therapeutic perspective but also from legal aspects. The fast investigation regarding identification, dosage and route of administration of the poison helps in better application of therapeutic measures. Saving the patient's life is a physician's prime concern; additionally, the purpose of poisoning - whether accidental, suicidal or homicidal - should be investigated.

Table 2.1 The Diagnosis of Poison in Living can be Done by:

| | | |
|---|---|---|
| 1. | History taking: | What did the person have for food. Whether there is symptom onset in others who had the same food. Diarrhoea and vomiting in mass of people. Whether there is consumption of suspicious foods. |

| 2. | Symptoms: | System wise symptoms:<br>• Ocular system: Blurry vision, dilated pupil, diplopia, photophobhia.<br>• Ears: Vertigo, deafness, tinnitus.<br>• Skin: Erythema, rashes, itching, hypothermia, hyperthermia.<br>• GI system: Vomiting, diarrhoea, constipation, melena, abdominal distention, abdominal pain, dysphagia.<br>• Excretory system: Polyuria, oliguria, burning micturition, Hematuria.<br>• CVS: Hypertension, hypotension, arrhythmia, tachycardia, bradycardia.<br>Respiratory system: Dyspnoea, coughing, bronchitis, pulmonary oedema. |
|---|---|---|
| 3. | Examinations: | • Diagnosis of barbiturates by cobaltous acetate, 5% iso-propylamine solutions. These tests prove the presence of suspected poisons in poisoned material. Hallucinogenic drugs like LSD are easily detected under ultra- violet light. Many alkaloids can be detected by chemical reactions.<br>• Chromatography screening.<br>• Thin layer chromatography.<br>• Liquid chromatography.<br>• Gas liquid chromatography.<br>• High liquid chromatography.<br>• Ultraviolet visible spectroscopy.<br>• Atomic absorption spectroscopy.<br>• Trace metal analyser.<br>• Breath alcohol analyser. |

- **Acute poisoning:** Manifestation of signs & symptoms is within a short time and attains complicated features. General symptoms of acute poisoning:

Vomiting, diarrhoea, convulsions, fainting, acute colic, borborygni, excessive salivation, deformed pupils, buzzing in the ears, hyperthermia, sweating, delirium, neurological symptoms, bluish discolouration, anxiety, respiratory distress, coldness of body-parts, restlessness.

- **Chronic poisoning:** Signs & symptoms develop gradually and at times remain concealed. Sometimes the course of chronic poisoning is so slow that its signs & symptoms represent themselves very mildly or as symptoms of another disease. Due to the mildness, diagnosis of chronic poisoning is completely missed. Common symptoms of chronic poisoning:

Restlessness, anxiety, weakness, loss of weight, On & off presentation of gastro-intestinal symptoms.

**1. The diagnosis of poison in dead can be done by:**
Medico-legal aspects are to be considered thoroughly in all deaths due to poisoning. Any unnatural death should be investigated for poisoning by various methods.

***A. Post-mortem examination:***

- **External examination:** Mark of vomitus and faeces, mark of injection, odours coming from mouth, external orifices for any stain, lividity like **cherry red colour: Carbon monoxide or brick red colour: cyanide**.

Table 2.2 External Examination

| Arsenic | Garlicky smell. |
|---|---|
| Cyanide | Bitter almond. |
| Ethyl alcohol | Fruity smell. |
| Cannabis | Burnt rope. |
| Hydrogen sulphide | Rotten eggs. |

Table 2.3 Internal Examination:

| GI tract | Poisonous contents like tablet, powder may be present. |
|---|---|
| Respiratory tract | Congestion of trachea, bronchi, lungs on inhaling poison. |
| Thickening and softening of wall | Corrosive and irritant poison. |
| Hard wall | Carbolic acid. |
| Perforation | H2SO4, HN3. |
| Leathery wall | Formaldehyde. |

***B. Chemical examination:***

Table 2.4 Routine viscera

| **Routine viscera:** | **Quantity:** |
|---|---|
| • Blood | 5 – 10 ml. |
| • Kidney | One half of each kidney. |
| • Stomach. | Entire. |
| • Stomach contents | 250 – 300 ml. |
| • Urine | 150 – 200 ml. |
| • Small intestine | Entire in infants.<br>100 cm in adults. |

Table 2.5 Specific viscera

| Specific Viscera: | Quantity: |
|---|---|
| • CSF: Alcohol poisoning | As much possible. |
| • Spinal cord: Kupilu poison | Whole length. |
| • Lung: Inhaled poison | Whole lung. |
| • Brain: Alcohol, barbiturate | One hemisphere. |

***C. Laboratory examination:***

Chromatography screening, thin layer chromatography, liquid chromatography, gas liquid chromatography, high liquid chromatography, ultraviolet visible spectroscopy, atomic absorption spectroscopy, trace metal analyser, breath alcohol analyser.

- **Vishaakta Achikitsya Lakshana:** Such patients should be rejected for treatment when poisoning case occurs.(सु. क. ३/४०–४४)

Table 2.6 Vishaakta Achikitsya Lakshana

| | |
|---|---|
| शस्त्रक्षते न रक्तं | No blood flow when cut by sharp instrument. |
| राज्योलताभिश्च न सम्भवन्ति | No body mark develops on tying with creepers. |
| शीताभी न रोमहर्ष | No horripilation on touching cold water. |
| सीत जिह्वा | Tongue becomes white. |
| केश शात | Hair fall occurs. |
| नासा कण्ठ भग्न | Nose and throat become broken. |
| कृष्ण सरक्त स्वयथु | Black reddish swelling. |
| हनु स्थिरत्व | Lower jaw doesn't move. |
| वर्ति घनास्य निरेति वक्त्रं | Thread like structure comes out from mouth. |

| रक्तं सृवेद उर्ध्वं अधः | Blood comes out from upper and lower orifices. |
|---|---|
| दम्स्ट्रानिपात | Bitten all over the body. |
| हीनस्वर | Low and insignificant voice. |
| विवर्णता | Discoloration. |

## 2.2 Chaturvimshati Upakrama:

"मन्त्रारिष्टोत्कर्तननिष्पीडनचूषणाआग्निपरिषेकौः।
अवगाहरक्तमोक्षणवमनविरेकोपधानानी।।३५।।
हृदयावरणाञ्जननस्यधूमलेहौषधप्रशमनानी।
प्रतिसारणं प्रतिविषं सञ्ज्ञासंस्थापनं लेपः।।३६।।
मृतसञ्जीवनमेव च विंशतिरेते चतुर्भिरधिकाः।
स्युरुपक्रमा यथा ये यत्र योज्याः श्रुणु तथा तान।।३७।।"
(च – चि– २३ / ३५–३७)

उपक्रमः Treatment

01) मन्त्र (Chanting of Mantra):

मंत्रस्य विषहरेषु श्रेष्ठत्वादग्रे अभिधानं। (च. चि. २३)

Mantra is mentioned first among all the upakrama as it brings down the effect of poison very soon. It is the combination of words which are pure and it helps the person to connect with the almighty. Mantra have the immense power to cure poison when recited with pure heart. While chanting mantra one should avoid all the types of tamasic activities and also sleep on sacred grass. While chanting mantra one should also worship the idol of God.

02) अरिष्ट बन्धन (Tourniquet):

दंशात्तु विषं दष्टस्याविसृतं वेणिकां भिषग्बद्ध्वा। (च. चि. २३)

As mentioned in Charak samhita indriya sthaana that arishta means which denotes end of life. When poison has increased to a significant level it shows arishta. This spread should be stopped as early as possible and so the physician has to tie a bandhan which can arrest the spread of poison. It can be tied by a tourniquet and if it is not available the cloth piece, rope, thread can also be used. If the bandhan is too tight it will lead to foul smelling at the site of bite and if it is too loose will continue the spread of arishta.

03) उत्कर्तन (Small incisions):

तरुरिव मूलच्छेदाददंशच्छेदान्न वृद्धिमेति विषं।। (च. चि. २३)

It is the process of incision of wound. When the pipe in which water flows is cut from a site the water doesn't flow, in the similar way when wound is incisioned, the blood will oose out and will not spread in the body.

04) निष्पीडन (Squeezing):

निष्पीड़यति निषपीड़नेन विषं गालयते। (च. चि. २३)

Nishpidan means squeezing. The process to remove poison from the site of bite by squeezing is called as nishpidan. When incision not done can do this procedure.

05) चूषण (Sucking):

This is the process to suck the poison out of the site where poison is located in fleshy parts. The mouth should first be filled with mud or cow dung like substance and then sucking process be done.

06) अग्निकर्म (Thermal cauterization):

For removal of visha located in Twaka and Mamsa. As Agni increases pitta Dosha it is contra indicated in pitta predominance. Just as fire applied to dry grass converts everything into ash in no time similarly this process also removes poison within seconds. When the bite is of mandali sarpa this method of removing poison is contra indicated.

07) परिषेक (Effusion):

The effusion is prepared by using cooling drugs like Chandana and Ushira. This should be made into decoction form and this decoction should be sprinkled over the poisoned part. This due to its cooling property condenses the poison and decreases its intensity. Acharya Charak has also mentioned the application of paste on the site of poison to decrease the intensity of poison.

08) अवगाह (Therapeutic bath):

The process of immersion of poisoned part into the medicated decoction is called as Avagaha. This may be done by a bath in decoction, sponging the decoction or by holding ice pack on the head.

09) रक्तमोक्षण (Blood letting):

विषं स्त्रावणं हरति रक्तात। (च. चि. २३)

The most important procedure to remove poison from the body. Blood is the most supportive media for poison to spread and so this is an effective methods to decrease the spread of poison. If the poisoned body is stiff, discolored, swollen then this procedure should be performed immediately. It is carried out around the vein at the site of bite.

10) वमन (Emesis):

पीतंवमनैः सध्योहरेत विरेकैरर्दवितीये तु। (च. चि. २३)

This helps in immediate removal of poison. During this the drugs having Vishaghna properties are used. When there are Kapha pre dominance and in Hemant Rutu then Tikshna Vamana Aushadhi should be given. This is the best method to remove the unabsorbed poison from the stomach. During administration of Vamana it should be kept in mind that any type of Kapha aggravating drugs like Kullatha should not be used.

11) विरेचन (Purgation):

This procedure should be done when the poison is in pakwashaya. When there is pain and burning abdomen, distension of abdomen, retention of urine, flatus, faeces this procedure should be done. According to Ashtang Sangraha this procedure should be done but avoiding the frequent getting up by the patient as this causes Vata aggravating and thus a bed pan should be given to the patient.

12) उपधान (Medication on incised scalp):

उपधानं विश्संकमणार्थ मस्तके भेषजादानाम। (च. चि. २३)

When due to the Kapha aggravating properties of poison obstruction is caused in channels than patient feels breathlessness and this can be fatal and so the incision is made on head of the shape of Kakapada(feet of crow) and one Bilva quantity paste of meat of goat, cow, buffalo should be applied on head which absorbs all the poison from body and helps in recovering.

13) हृदयावरण (Protection of heart):

आदौ हृदयं रक्ष्यं तस्यावरणं पिबेध्यथलाभं।
मधुसर्पिर्मज्जपयोगैरिकमथ गोमयरसं वा।।

Heart is the most vital organ of body. So in case of poisoning it should be protected first. Honey, Ghrita, bone marrow, milk, Gairik, cow dung, sugarcane juice should be mixed and be used for the protection of heart. In case of severe poisoning the heart should be protected first and so modern has also mentioned it as cardio protective drugs. Ingestion of drugs soon after poisoning helps to decrease the speed of spread of poison.

14) अञ्जन (Collyrium):

If there is obstruction of eyes then Anjana should be given. Devdaru, Karveera, Maricha, Nimba, Pippali should be triturated and made into a paste by mixing with Gomutra and should be applied over the eyes. Anjana should be performed as according to Acharya Vagbhatt opines that the penetrating quality of poison causes dryness in eyes.

15) नस्य (Nasal medication):

शिरोगते विषे मूलंनस्यकर्मणियोजयेत।

Bharangi, Pippali, Hingu, Manahshila, Shirisha beeja, Apamarga, Lavana should be made into powder and be used as Pradhaman Nasya. When the poison reaches head nasal medication as mentioned above should be used.

नासाक्षि कर्ण जिह्वा कण्ठ निरोधेषु कर्म नस्त स्यात।

If there is obstruction in nose, eyes, ears, throat then Nasya should be done. This is also used to cure the local symptoms like headache, heaviness of head.

16) धूमन (Medical smoking):

This process helps to clear the channels and also helps to nullify the effect of poison. The drugs which give antiseptic action are used for Dhuman at local site of bite. The drugs are taken in a vessel and are heated and the smoke coming out is used which decrease the effect of poison. According to Acharya Sushruta wherever Swedan is contra indicated there Dhuman is also contra indicated. Also in Vrushchika Damsh Dhuman is contra indicated.

17) लेह (Linctus):

Lehan means to lick. The medicine which can be licked is called as Lehya. When poison is intaken due to the Ruksha, Ushna Guna of poison the mouth and throat gets dried this is a situation where patient cannot drink any medicine and so Lehan should be done of anti-poisonous drugs. Lehya preparation are mostly of Ghrita and Madhu combination.

18) औषध (Anti-poisonous drugs):

In case of poisoning medicine should be given internally. Poison aggravates a particular Dosha in body and so medicine should be given accordingly which are opposite Guna of poison. The drugs which can be given are Mruta Sanjivani yoga, Agad yoga.

19) प्रशमन (Sedatives):

After the proper Snehan and Swedan some Dosha are still remaining in the body and if these dosha are not eliminated than it may lead to death. So Lepa like procedure should be done.

20) प्रतिसारण (Application of alkalies):

This is also called as Pragharshan. While Raktamokshan process if blood doesn't come out than dry drugs such as Trikatu, Haridra are used to rub over the site. This decreases extra moisture, itching and effects of poison.

21) प्रतिविष (Antidotes):

विषे प्रतिविषं योज्यं मन्त्रैतंत्रैरसिध्यति ।
अतीते पंचमे वेगे सप्तमस्यानतीक्रमे ।।

When the poisonous effect doesn't subside by any medicine or procedure than its antidote should be given. It should be given when 5th stage ends. It should be administered according to kala. But in emergency can be administered anytime. Sthavara visha spreads upward and Jangama visha spreads downward and so they act as antidote for each other.

22) संज्ञास्थापन (Resuscitation):

This helps for regaining the consciousness of a person. When a person lies with loss of Sanjna and has neck hanging should be done Shirovirechan. Also when patient recovers then Shodhan should be done.

23) लेप (Local application of medicines):

When the roots of a tree are cut its growth decreases automatically. In a similar manner when at the site of bite application of Lepa made of Shita virya drugs and anti poison properties are applied it decreases the effect of poison very effectively.

24) मृतसञ्जीवन (Revival):

This is the classical method by which the life of an individual can be regained. This procedure can be used for nullification of any type of poison. This method prevents the ultimate death.

Image 2.1 Image for gastric lavage

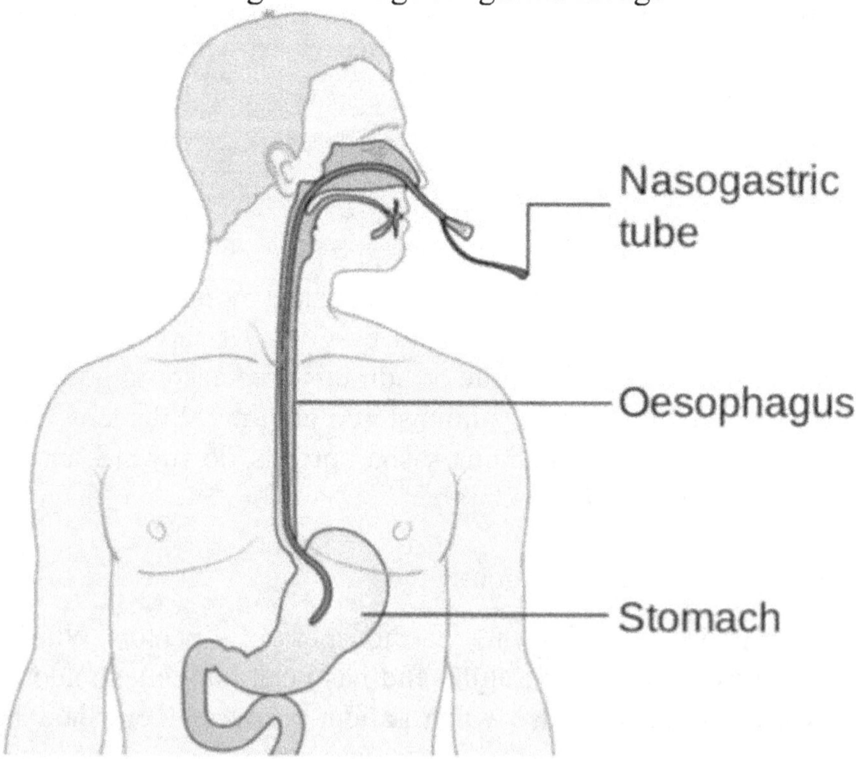

## 2.3 General Principles for Management of Poisoning:

Table 2.7 General Principles for Management of Poisoning

| | |
|---|---|
| • Stabilization | • A: Airway.<br>• B: Breathing.<br>• C: Circulation.<br>• D: Depression of CNS.<br>• When there is normal pulse then thorough complete examination be done.<br>• For comatose patients, 3 antidotes – Dextrose 5% 100 ml IV + Thiamine 100 ml IV + Naloxone 2mg IV. |
| • Gut decontamination | • Emesis: Done by common salt, mustard, IPECAC. It activates CTZ and should be done 4-6 hours of poison ingestion.<br>• Gastric lavage: Emptying the stomach from toxic substances. Should be done within 1-2 hours of poison ingestion. In drugs like salicylate, it can be useful upto 12-16 hours.<br>• In adults, 30 to 40 French Ewald tube is useful.<br>• In children, 16 to 28 Ryle's tube is useful.<br>• Material used are Warm water, NS. |
| • Antidotes | • These are called as Magic Bullets which counter the adverse effects of poison immediately.<br>• Mechanical antidote: Bulky food like glass powder, egg albumin, charcoal dust.<br>• Chemical antidote: Weak alkalies for strong acid poisons, weak acids for strong alkalies.<br>• Physostigmine for atropine poisoning.<br>• Nalorphine for morphine poisoning.<br>• BAL: For arsenic, gold, mercury, bismuth, other heavy metals. |
| • Catharsis | • Relief provided from poison by inducing purgation.<br>• Materials: Saline, Saccharides. |
| • Activated charcoal | • Absorbs the poison on its surface, there by decreasing the absorption of poison in gut.<br>• Adult dose: 50-100 gm.<br>• Child dose: 10-30 gm. |
| • Whole bowel irrigation | • Large amount of solution is instilled by nasogastric tube for 2-6 hours. This causes diarrhoea.<br>• Done by PEG – ELS, PEG – 3350. |
| • Symptomatic treatment | • Trendelenburg position be given to the patient.<br>• When extreme gut problems, electrolyte replacement should be done. |

## 2.4 Duties of Medical Practitioner in Case of Suspected Poisoning:

- Prompt diagnosis of the poison. Care & treatment of the patient in case of doubt, the physician should stick to general line of treatment and manage the patient symptomatically.
- Taking care of legal proceedings. The physician should note the name, address, sex, age, occupation, date & time of arrival, accompanying members and complete history of the patient. In case of a dying patient, the dying declaration should be noted immediately.
- In case of sudden or accidental poisoning, if the physician feels that there can be a mass poisoning, then he should promptly inform the concerned authorities about the same.
- In case of suspected homicidal poisoning, the physician should immediately consult an expert Toxicologist and Forensic Science experts.
- On confirmation of homicidal poisoning, the physician should inform the police and other concerned authorities.
- The patient should be immediately removed from the location of poisoning and it is always judicious to admit him in a hospital.
- All the documents and evidences carefully preserved. Gastric contents, vomitus, faecal matter, blood samples, etc. should be stored in containers and appropriately labelled.
- If the patient dies, death certificate must not be issued.
- In case of poisoning, medical officers of Government and public hospitals should immediately inform the legal authorities.

**Multiple Choice Questions:**

**1.Which of the following is not a symptom for ocular poisoning?**

A. Diplopia B. Blurred vision C. Arrhythmias D. Photophobhia

**2.What is the dose of activated charcoal in child?**
A. 60mg B. 10mg C. 90mg D. 45mg

**3.For chemical examination, in routine viscera what is the amount of urine collected?**
A. 150ml B. 50ml C. 1Ltr D. 300ml

**4.What is the synonym for antidote?**
A. Revival B. Magic bullets C. Catharsis D. Homicide

5. ________ विश्संकमणार्थ मस्तके भेषजादानाम। (च. चि. २३) **is the Shloka for which Upakrama?**

A. अंजन B. नस्य C. उपधान D. वमन

**6. Burnt rope smell comes from which poisoning?**
A. Morphine B. Mercury C. Gold D. Cannabis

**7.In routine viscera, what is the amount of blood collected for chemical examination?**
A. 10ml B. 20ml C. 17ml D. 1ml

**8. Whole bowel irrigation is done by which substance?**
A. IPECAC B. Mustard C. PEG – ELS D. Common salt

**9. Manifestation of signs & symptoms is within a short time and attains complicated features. Shows which type of poisoning?**
A. Chronic B. Acute C. Subacute D. Fulminant

10. पीतंवमनैः सध्योहरेत विरेकैरर्दवितीये तु। (च. चि. २३) **is the Shloka for which Upakrama?**

A. वमन B. रक्तमोक्षण C. विरेचन D. परिषेक

**11.What is the size of French Ewald tube used for gut decontamination in adults?**

A. 16 to 28 B. 35 to 45 C. 10 to 15 D. 30 to 40

**12.What is not the type of poisoning?**

A. Primary B. Accidental C. Suicidal D. Homicidal

**13.Which poisonous material has a garlicky smell?**

A. Cyanide B. Arsenic C. Ethyl alcohol D. Hydrogen sulphide

**14. Which of the following is not a specific viscera?**

A. CSF B. Spinal cord C. Kidney D. Lung

**15. British Anti Lewisite is not an antidote for which poisoning?**

A. Gold B. Atropine C. Mercury D. Bismut

**Answer key for MCQs:**

| | |
|---|---|
| 1 | C |
| 2 | B |
| 3 | A |
| 4 | B |
| 5 | C |
| 6 | D |
| 7 | A |
| 8 | C |

| | |
|---|---|
| 9 | B |
| 10 | C |
| 11 | D |
| 12 | A |
| 13 | B |
| 14 | C |
| 15 | B |

# Ch. 3
# Vishakta Ahara Pariksha and Viruddha Ahara

## 3.1 Sources of exposure of Visha with Contemporary Relevance

अन्ने पाने दन्तकाष्ठे तथा अभ्यंगे अवलेखने।
उत्सादने कषाये च परिषेके अनुलेपने।।
स्त्रक्षु वस्त्रेषु शय्यासु कवचाभरणेषु च।
पादुकापादपीठेषु पृष्ठेषु गजवाजिनाम्।।
विषजुष्टेषु चान्येषु नरयधूग अंजनादिषु।
लक्ष्णानि प्रवक्ष्यामि चिकित्सामप्यनन्तरम्।। (सु.क. १/ २५–२६)

It can be due to infliction of poison in food and drinks, toothbrush, oil or paste for massaging, garlands, dress, bed sheets, footwear, covers on back of elephant or horse, Nasya, Dhuma, Anjana.

- In the present era, adulterated foods and unhealthy packing materials are the main source for illness.
- The use of over the counter medicines can cause poisoning specifically the drugs which are addictive in nature.
- Due to use of fruits and vegetables grown by pesticides. Use of chemicals to grow fruits faster and giving artificial sweetness.
- Due to use of fruits and vegetables affected by pests or worms.
- Excess use of micro flours and its preparation like pizza, burger, etc. junk foods.
- Milk is nowadays prepared to sell by mixing urea to increase the amount of profit.
- Clostridium botulinum which can develop in vacuum-packaged and canned foods and Listeria monocytogenes occurs due to improper cleaning of food preparation machines.

- Raw meat may contain harmful bacteria including Salmonella, Campylobacter and E.coli that can cause food poisoning. These bacteria are destroyed when meat is correctly cooked.

**Water pollution:** A major source of water pollution is runoff from agricultural fields, industrial sites, or urban areas. Run-off disrupts the water body's natural balance.

- For example, agricultural run-off typically includes fertilizer or toxic chemicals. Fertilizer can cause algal blooms (an explosive growth of algae).
- Choking out other plants and decreasing the amount of available oxygen necessary for the survival of other species. Raw sewage is another type of water pollutant.
- When sewage gets into the drinking water supply, serious stomach and digestive issues may result, including the spread of diseases such as typhoid or dysentery.
- A third source of water pollution is trash. Improperly disposed of items, such as plastic bags, fishing line, and other materials may accumulate in the water and lead to the premature death of animals that get tangled within the garbage.

**Soil pollution:** Soil can become polluted by industrial sources or the improper disposal of toxic chemical substances.

- Common sources of soil pollution include asbestos, lead, PCBs, and overuse of pesticides or herbicides.
- Additionally, various compounds get into the soil from the atmosphere, for instance with precipitation water, as well as by wind activity or other types of soil disturbances, and from surface water bodies and shallow groundwater flowing through the soil.
- Humans can be affected by soil pollution through the inhalation of gases emitted from soils moving upward, or through the inhalation of matter that is disturbed and transported by the wind because of the various human activities on the ground.

- Soil pollution may cause a variety of health problems, starting with headaches, nausea, fatigue, skin rash, eye irritation and potentially resulting in more serious conditions like neuromuscular blockage, kidney and liver damage and various forms of cancer.

**Air pollution:** A major source of air pollution results from the burning of fossil fuels.

- The Vehicle and factory emissions are common sources of this type of air pollution. The burning of fossil fuels contributes to the formation of smog, a dense layer of particulate matter that hangs like a cloud over many major cities and industrial zones.
- Air pollution contributes to respiratory problems such as asthma, lung cancer, chronic bronchitis, and other lung ailments.
- Nitrogen and sulphur oxides in the air contribute to acid rain, which is a form of precipitation with a lower (more acidic) pH than normal.
- Acid rain harms forests, species that live in water bodies, and degrades outdoor statues, monuments, and buildings.

### 3.2 Vishakta Ahara Pariskha

- ***Methods for the diagnosis of Visha are as follows:***

1. Agniparikshana
2. Panchbhautika Parikshana
3. Pariksha of animals and birds
4. Bhautika Parikshana
5. Lakshananusara Parikshana

a. Lakshana of Sthavara and Jangama Visha
b. Lakshana according to mode of administration
c. Lakshana according to site of poison
d. Lakshana according to use of poisoned material
e. Lakshana of Garvisha & Dooshivisha

6. Ashrumrut parikshana

***1. Agniparikshana:*** Poisoned materials burn with single point flame (not with normal spreading flame), become like peacock's neck, interrupted and slow emit flames of different colours like rainbow, and gives out cracking sound. The emerged smoke has cadaveric smell.

***2. Indriya Parikshana:***

Table 3.1 Indriya parikshana for poison

| | |
|---|---|
| Shabda Parikshana | poisoned food burns making loud cracks. |
| Sparsha Parikshana | contact with poisoned food causes burning sensation and nails falling of hands. |
| Rupa Parikshana | when cast into the fire, poisoned material acquires the colours of peacock's neck. |
| Rasa Parikshana | lack of its natural taste |
| Gandha Parikshana | on burning poisoned material emits irritating fumes which smells like a cadaver. |

***3. Pariksha of Animals and Birds:*** Voice of Kokila (cuckoo) changed, gait of swan gets altered, Bhringraja bird (domestic crane) becomes excited, Karkavaku (cock) hoots loudly, Suka (green parakeet) and Sarika (mynah) makes long loud sounds. Chamikara vomits. Karandava (white breasted goose) fly away. Birds either die or faint. Nakula (moongoose) gets horripilation. Vanara (monkey) eliminates faeces. Prushta (spotted deer) weeps. Mayoora (peacock) gets elated.

### *4. Bhautika Parikshana:*

Table 3.2 Examination for poisoned foods & liquids

| | |
|---|---|
| Poisoned foods | • Food mixed with poison requires long time to cook. And cooked food becomes stale.<br>• Loses its natural odour, colour, smell, taste.<br>• Becomes very moist and appears to be full of glistening particles.<br>• Poisoned materials burn with single point flame. |
| Poisoned liquids | • Kvatha becomes dark, black or blue coloured.<br>• Poisoned water gets distorted.<br>• Mirror images don't appear.<br>• Accumulation of foams.<br>• Blue lines in Mamsa rasa, copper lines in milk, black lines in alcohol, brown lines in ghee, red lines in oil |

### *5. Lakshanusara Pariksha:*

Table 3.3 Lakshana of Sthavara and Jangama Visha

| | |
|---|---|
| Sthavara Visha | Jvara, Hikka, Dantaharsha, Galagraha, Phena, Vamana, Aruchi, Shvasa, Murccha. |
| Jangama Visha | Nidra, Tandra, Klama, Daha, Paka, Lomaharshana, Shopha, Atisara. |

Table 3.4 Lakshana according to poison administration

| | |
|---|---|
| Vishdhuma (poisonous fumes) | Inhalation of poisonous fumes or smoke causes fainting, watering of eyes and mouth, headache, running nose and disturbances of the vision. |
| Vapour of poisoned food | Cardiac pain, abnormal movement of eyes and headache. |
| Vishjushta dantkashta (poisoned tooth brush) | Causes dryness and swelling of palate, teeth, tongue and lips. |

| | |
|---|---|
| Vishjushta anjana (poisoned collyrium) | Application causes accumulation of dirt in eyes, redness, pain, distortion of vision and even blindness. |
| Vishjushta nasyamdhum (poisoned snuff and smoke) | Causes headache, discharge of Kapha (watery fluid), bleeding through the natural orifices (nose, mouth and eyes). |
| Poisoned ear drops | Causes swelling, pain, ulcers and defects of hearing. |
| Smelling poisoned flowers | Causes headache, tears in the eyes and loss of sensation of smell. |

Table 3.5 Lakshana according to site of Poison

| | |
|---|---|
| Visha in mouth (ingestion) | Causes tingling sensation in lips, burning sensation inside the mouth, hardness at the root of tongue, lockjaw, more salivation, loss of sensation of taste, pricking pain. |
| Visha in Amashaya (poisoned food in stomach) | Causes perspiration, toxicity, fainting, vomiting, discolouration, distention of abdomen, burning sensation, loss of appetite, appearance of rashes (spots) all over the body. Flatulence, trembling and abnormality of sense organs. |
| Visha in Pakvashaya (poisoned food in intestine) | Causes thirst, burning sensation, fainting, diarrhoea, gurgling noise in the abdomen, stupor, loss of strength, emaciation, pallor and enlargement of the abdomen. |

Table 3.6 Lakshana according to use of poisoned material

| | |
|---|---|
| Vishjushta Taila (poisoned oil) | Used for oil bath produce burning sensation in the skin, perspiration, ulcers, bleed and lacerations. |
| Poisoned oil for application on head | Produce headache, appearance of nodules, and falling of hairs. |

| | |
|---|---|
| Poisoned comb | Causes falling of hair, headache, bleeding from passage and appearance of cysts on head. |
| Poisoned wooden foot wear | Causes inflammation, discharge, numbness, and eruption of boils in feet. |
| Poisoned ornaments | Causes burning sensation, suppuration and tearing of poisoned material. |

Table 3.7 Lakshana of Garavisha & Dooshivisha

| | |
|---|---|
| Garavisha (artificially mixed poison) | Garavisha is prepared by mixing more than a single poisonous or non-poisonous drugs. It may produce swelling, anaemia, enlargement of abdomen, insanity, piles etc. |
| Dooshivisha (weak/chronic poison) | This is the weak and latent poison. One suffering from Dooshivisha passes liquid stool of abnormal colour, has foul smell, tasteless sensation in mouth, thirst, fainting, vomiting and other symptoms of toxicity. |

**6. Ashrumrut Pariksha:**

- External and internal findings (sings) confirms the diagnosis of poisoning. For the homicidal purpose, poison was ingested with mixing in food materials. Black coloured hands, legs, teeth and nails in the dead body confirms it.
- Improper posture, scattered cloths and the number of episodes of diarrhoea occurred confirms death by Dhatura poisoning.
- Discharge of blood from bite site, indicates snake bite.
- Food materials found in the dead was subjected to birds for the confirmation of the poisoning.

- **Visha Data Lakshana:**

Visha Data Lakshana are the features of the person who intends to poison or poisoned food, drinks, etc.

***A) According to Charaka Samhita***

अत्यर्थशन्कितः स्याद बहुवागथवाल्पवाग्विगतलक्ष्मीः।
प्राप्तः प्रकृति विकारं विषप्रदाता नरो ज्ञेयः।। (च.चि.२३–१०७)

A person who behaves in an extremely suspicious manner, who is garrulous or who speaks very little, who has lost lustre of his face and who exhibits changes in his characteristics is a poison-giver (Visha Data).

***B) According to Sushruta Samhita:***

यसमाच्च चेतोअनित्यत्वमश्ववत् प्रथितं नृणम् ।
न विश्वस्यात्ततो राजा कदाचिदपि कस्यचित् ।। (सु.क.१)

The intelligent physician who can understand the intention of others by their speech, action and facial expressions should recognize the person who puts poison (to foods, drinks, etc.) by the following features:

He who does not reply when questioned, becomes disillusioned while talking, speaks irrelevantly and enigmatically or like an idiot, makes sound with his fingers, scratches the ground, falls on the ground, trembles with fear, becomes thin, discoloured face, tears something with his nails, pulls his hair often, tries to go out through the wrong door, looks around again and again, behaves in all opposite manners and becomes unconscious

***C) According to Ashtanga Hridaya:***

विषदः श्याव शुष्कास्यो विलक्षो वीक्षते दिशः।
स्वेद वेपथु मांस्त्रस्तो भीतः स्खलति जृम्भते।। (अ.हृ.सू.७–१२)

The face of the person who has maliciously poisoned food will be dark, his mouth will be dry, he will look aimlessly here and there, he will sweat profusely, shiver, remain stupefied with fear, stumbles while walking, stammers and yawns frequently.

### 3.3 Adulteration and Tests for its Detection

An adulterant is a chemical substance which should not be contained within other substances (e.g. food, beverages, and fuels) for legal or other reasons.

- The addition of adulterants : adulteration.
- The word is appropriate only when the additions are unwanted by the recipient.

Otherwise the expression would be food additive.

- Adulterants when used in illicit drugs are called cutting agents.
- **Food is said to be adulterated if:**
- The article sold by a vendor is not of the nature, substance or quality demanded by the purchaser.
- The article contains any other substance which affects the nature, substance or quality.
- Any inferior or cheaper substance has been substituted.
- The article had been prepared, packed or kept under insanitary conditions whereby

it has become contaminated or injurious to health.

- The article consists wholly or in part of any filthy, putrid, rotten, decomposed or diseased animal or vegetable substance or is insect-infested or is otherwise unfit for human consumption.
- The article is obtained from a diseased animal.
- The article contains any poisonous or other ingredient which renders it injurious to health.
- The container of the article is composed of any poisonous or deleterious substance which renders its contents injurious to health.
- Any colouring matter other than that prescribed is present in the article.
- The article contains any prohibited preservative or permitted preservative in excess of the prescribed limits.

Table 3.8 Different Types of Food Adulteration:

| | |
|---|---|
| Intentional | Sand, marble chips, stones, mud, other filth, talc, chalk powder, water, mineral oil |
| Incidental | Pesticide residues tin from can, droppings of rodents, larvae in foods. |
| Metallic contamination | Arsenic from pesticides, lead from water, mercury from effluent, from chemical industries, tins from cans. |
| Packaging Hazards | Polyethylene, polyvinyl chloride and allied compounds are used to produce flexible packaging material |

Table 3.9 Some Adulterated Foods

| **Substances** | **Adulterant** | **Health hazards** |
|---|---|---|
| Turmeric, dals and pulses | Metanil, Yellow and Kesari Dal. | Highly carcinogenic, stomach disorders. |
| Green chilies, green peas & other vegetable | Malachite Green, Argemone seeds. | Carcinogenic if consumed over a long period of time. |
| Mustard seeds and mustard oil | Argemone seeds, Papaya seeds. | Epidemic dropsy and severe glaucoma. |
| Paneer, khoya, condensed milk and milk | Starch and water. | Stomach disorder. |
| Ice cream | Pepperonil, Ethylacetate, Butraldehyde, Nitrate, Washing powder, etc | Pepperonil is used as a pesticide and ethyl acetate causes diseases affecting lungs, kidneys and heart. |
| Coffee powder | Tamarind seeds, chicory powder. | Diarrhoea, stomach disorders, giddiness and severe joint pain. |

*Some other adulterants:*

- Cream is adulterated with gelatine, and formaldehyde is employed as a preservative for it.
- Butter is adulterated to an enormous extent with oleomargarine, a product of beef fat.
- Brick dust in chili powder, coloured chalk powder in turmeric.
- In confectionery, dangerous colours, such as chrome yellow, Prussian blue, copper and arsenic compounds are employed.
- Pickles and canned vegetables are sometimes coloured green with copper salts.

- Tests for detecting adulteration:

***a) Milk:*** Detection of water in milk:

Put a drop of milk on a polished slanting surface. Pure milk either stays or flows slowly leaving a white trail behind. Milk adulterated with water will flow immediately without leaving a mark.

***b) Honey:***

Take a tablespoon of honey and put it in a glass of water. If the honey dissolves, then it is not pure. Pure honey should stay together as a solid when submerged in water.

***c) Coconut oil:***

Coconut solidifies when cooled and this property can be used to check the adulteration of other oils in it. Take a transparent glass and keep in the refrigerator. After a few hours, the coconut layer will solidify and there will be a separate layer if it has adulteration of other oils.

## 3.4 Techniques used in the Detection of Poisons

Table 3.10 Tests for the detection of poison

| Test | Procedure | Result |
|---|---|---|
| Trinder's test | 2ml urine is taken and 100ml trinder's reagent is added. Mix for 5 seconds. | Violet colour shows presence of salicylate. |
| Gerrard's test | 1-2 ml of 2% mercuric chloride solution in 50% of alcohol is added to a portion of residue of the extract. A red colour develops immediately. | Hyoscyamine produces a yellow colour which becomes red on burning, while hyoscine does not produce any change of colour. |
| Fujiwara test | Dilute 1ml of sample with 2ml of sodium hydroxide solution. Add 2ml ferrous sulphate solution. Add sufficient hydrochloric acid to dissolve the ferrous hydroxide precipitate. | Blue colour indicates the presence of cyanide. |
| Marquis reagent test | Place a drop of marquis reagent (prepared by adding 3ml of conc. Sulphuric acid and 3 drops of formalin) on the suspected scene residue or add few drops to stomach contents. | A purple coloration which gradually turns into violet and finally to blue colour indicates the presence of opium and its derivatives. |
| FPN test | 5ml of ferric chloride solution, 45 ml of 20% solution of perchloric acid and 50 ml of 50% solution of nitric acid is added to make a final solution. | Colour ranging from pink to red, orange, violet or blue colour indicates presence of phenothiazines. |
| Duquenois levine test | Small amount of suspected residue of extract is placed in a test tube and shaken with 2ml.of a duquenois reagent for one minute and further 2ml of concentration. Hydrochloric acid is added, shaken and allowed to stand for 10 minutes. If a colour develops, 2ml of chloroform is added. | The violet coloured layer gives the positive indication of presence of cannabis. |

## 3.5 Viruddha Ahara with Contemporary Relevance

यत्किन्चिद्दोषमुत्क्लेश्य न हरेत्तत्समासतः विरुद्धं।। (अ.हृ.सू ७/४५)

- Any foods, drinks or drugs which aggravate the Doshas in body but do not expel them is called as viruddha ahara. The person who takes Viruddha-Ahara should be subjected to either Shodhana or Shamana karma with Dravya which have opposite Guna to the ingested Viruddha Ahara.

- ***According to*** चरक संहिता सुत्रस्थान (२६/६१–६२), ***types of Viruddha Ahara is:***

***1) Kanichit Paraspara Guna Viruddhani:***

Some substances act against the health due to their mutually contradictory qualities.

***2) Kanichit Samyogat:***

Some substances act against the health due to combination of 2 or more Dravyas.

***3) Samskarat:***

Some substances act against the health due to the method of preparation.

***4) Desha Kala Matradi:***

Some substances act against the health due to virtue of Desha, Kala & Matra.

***5) Svabhavat:***

Some substances act against the health due to their inherent nature.

Table 3.11 Viruddha Bheda: - Types: 18

| 1.Desha Viruddha | Intake of Ruksha & Tikshna Dravya in Jangala Desha.<br>Intake of Sheeta & Snigdha Dravya in Anupa Desha. |
|---|---|
| 2.Kala Viruddha | Intake of Sheeta & Ruksha Dravya in Sheeta Kala (Ritu).<br>Intake of Katu & Ushna Dravya in Ushna Kala (Ritu). |
| 3.Agni Viruddha | Intake of Guru Ahara in case of Mandagni.Intake of Laghu Ahara in case of Tikshnagni.<br>Irregular intake of Ahara in case of Vishama or Samagni. |

| 4.Matra Viruddha | Intake of Madhu & Ghrita in equal quantity. |
|---|---|
| 5.Satmya Viruddha | Intake of Madhura & Sheeta Ahara if accustomed to Katu & Ushna Ahara |
| 6.Dosha Viruddha | Ahara, Aushadha or Vihara similar to Dosha which are opposite the person's practice. |
| 7.Samskara Viruddha | Ahara and Aushadha prepared in a particular way which produces poisonous effect like Pippali prepared with Matsya and Kakamachi mixed with Madhu. |
| 8.Veerya Viruddha | Intake of Sheeta Veerya with Ushna Veerya Dravya. e.g.: Dugdha with Matsya |
| 9.Kostha Viruddha | Administration of Sukha - Virechana in a small dose for a person with Krura - Kostha; administration of Tikshna Virechana for a person with Mridu – Kostha. |
| 10.Avastha Viruddha | Intake of Vata aggravating Dravya in case of Shrama or after Vyayama or Vyavaya.<br>Intake of Kapha aggravating Dravya in case of Ati - Nidra or Alasya. |
| 11.Krama Viruddha | Intake of Ahara before his bowel or urinary bladder is clear. Intake of Ahara when there is no appetite or appetite is highly aggravated. |
| 12.Parihara Viruddha | Intake of Ushna Dravya after intake of pork, etc. |
| 13.Upachara Viruddha | Intake of Sheeta Dravya after intake of ghee, etc. |
| 14.Paka Viruddha | Intake of Ahara which is prepared with bad or rotten food, frozen food or preparation process includes excessive coldness or heat. |
| 15.Samyoga Viruddha | Caused by combination of 2 or more Dravya.The specific toxic properties are produced by combination of Dravyas, which cannot be manifested by the individual substance. E.g.: Dugdha with Amla Dravya. |
| 16.Hridaya Viruddha | Intake of Ahara which is not pleasing to the Mana. |
| 17.Sampat Viruddha | Intake of Ahara which is not matured, over-matured or putrefied. |
| 18.Vidhi Viruddha | Intake of Ahara not according to Vidhi - Vidhana. E.g.: Intake of food in unhygienic place or while talking or laughing, etc. |

## 3.6 Food Poisoning and Amavisha

Food poisoning is characterized by a group of symptoms or illnesses caused by ingestion of contaminated, spoiled, or toxic food articles.

Table 3.12 Causative bacteria, symptoms & prevention of food poisoning

| Bacteria | Cause | Symptoms | Preventing methods |
|---|---|---|---|
| Botulinum | Improperly canned foods, garlic infused oils, honey. | Diplopia, blurred vision, musclc weakness, breathing problems. | Avoid food from leaky cans, boil canned food for 10 minutes. Store garlic infused oils in cold place. |
| E.coli | Contaminated water, raw milk, raw grounded beef, contaminated animal faeces contact. | Diarrhoea, bloody discharge, nausea, abdominal cramps. | Never drink unpasteurized milk, follow proper washroom hygiene. Avoid bare hands contact with animal faeces. |
| Listeria | Unpasteurized milk, uncooked meat. | Fever, chills, headache, backache, diarrhoea, abdominal cramps. | Avoid unpasteurized milk and cook meat at 70° C to 75° C. |
| Salmonella | Undercooked meat, poultry, eggs. Raw water or ice. | Diarrhoea, abdominal cramps, nausea, fever, chills, headache. | Avoid raw or undercooked meat or poultry. Use clean utensils and surfaces to cook. |

Table 3.13 Causative fishes, symptoms & prevention of food poisoning

| **Fishes** | **Symptoms** | **Prevention** |
|---|---|---|
| Tuna, mackerel | Burning around the mouth, diarrhoea, nausea, headache, palpitations, rashes. | Fishes should be stored in cool place, refrigerated immediately to avoid histamine formation |
| Shellfish | Burning around the mouth, fingers, toes, face. | Fishes caught during algal blooms should not be eaten. |

| Rudder fish | Oily diarrhoea, abdominal cramps, nausea, vomiting, headache. | Avoid eating fishes with high ester oil contents. |
|---|---|---|

- **Amavisha:**

  विरुद्धाध्यशनाजीर्णाशनशीलिन पुनरामदोषमामविषमित्याचक्षते भिषज।
  विषसदृशलिंगत्वात तत्त परमसाध्म्, आशुकारित्वादिरुद्धोपक्रमत्वाच्चेति।।
  (च. वि. २/१२)

Amavisha is the characteristic toxic features of indigestion. The person who is habituated to eat Viruddha ahara, Adhyashan and who eats during Ajirna has Amadosha which gets converted into Amavisha which is impossible to cure.

The symptoms of Amavisha are as follows:

| विष्टंभ | Doesn't like moving. |
|---|---|
| सदन | Physical and mental discomfort |
| शिरसो रुक | Headache |
| मूर्छा भ्रम | Unconsciousness, giddiness |
| पृष्ठ कटि ग्रह | Backache |
| जृम्भा | Yawning |
| अंगमर्द | Bodyache |
| तृष्णा | Thirst |
| ज्वर | Fever |
| छर्दि | Vomiting |
| अरोचक अविपाक | Anorexia, indigestion. |

- **Management of Ama pradosha:**
- When new initiation, then cured by giving Vamana by लवणोदक.
- In Vishuchika, give Langhan and then give Virechana.
- When patient has digested the previous meal but still has

heaviness of stomach than initially give Pachana and Deepan drugs to eliminate the remaining Doshas. When food given during this condition it worsens the state of disease.

- When all the Doshas are removed systematically then should be given Asthapan and Anuvasan Basti and diets should be followed as per Dosha, Satmya, Kala etc. factors affecting Agni. Apatarpan Chikitsa should also be followed.

**Multiple Choice Questions:**

**1. Which is not a method to diagnose Visha?**

A. Bhautik pariksha B. Agnipariksha

C. Vidhi pariksha D. Panchbhautika pariksha

**2. Which is a Sthavara Visha Lakshana?**

A. Nindra B. Tandra C. Klama D. Phena

**3. Green chillies are adulterated with which substance?**

A. Pepperonil B. Malachite green C. Metanil D. Chicory powder

**4. Severe glaucoma is caused due to adulteration in which substance?**

A. Mustard B. Turmeric C. Khoya D. Coffee pwder

**5. Trinder's test shows presence of which poisonous substance?**

A. Cyanide B. Opium C. Cannabis D. Salicylate

**6. Which is not a type of Viruddha Ahara?**

A. Lakshana B. Desha C. Agni D. Dosha

**7. FPN test is for which poisonous substance?**

A. Hyoscyamine B. Opium C. Phenothiazines D. Cannabis

**8. Rudder fish causes which type of diarrhoea?**

A. Watery B. Oily C. Bloody D. Mucus

**9.** विरुद्धाध्यशनाजीर्णाशनशीलिन पुनरामदोषमामविषमित्याचक्षते भिषज **….. is the Shloka for?**

A. Viruddha Ahara B. Sthavara Visha

C. Amavisha D. Jangama Visha

**10. Butter is adulterated to an enormous extent with which substance?**

A. Gelatin B. Oleomargarine C. Formaldehyde D. Copper salts

**Answer key for MCQs:**

| | |
|---|---|
| 1 | C |
| 2 | D |
| 3 | B |
| 4 | A |
| 5 | D |

| | |
|---|---|
| 6 | A |
| 7 | C |
| 8 | B |
| 9 | C |
| 10 | B |

# Ch. 4
# Garavisha and Dooshivisha

## 4.1 Garavisha

ग्र् + अच means to ingest. This means that the poison form is such that it can degluted. It can be made of combination of 2 poisonous or non poisonous substances.

नानाप्राण्यंगशमलविरुद्धौषधिभस्मनाम् ।
विषाणां चाल्पवीर्याणां योगो गर इति स्मृतः ।।
(अ.हृ.ऊ. ३५/४६–५०)

Different body organs of dead animals, excreta of animals, incompatible substances or drugs, ashes and poisonous substances with a lower potency can all be considered as Garavisha.

गरसंयोगजं चान्यद गरसंज्ञं गदप्रदम् ।
कालान्तरविपाकित्वान्न तदाशु हरत्यसून् ।। (च.चि.२३/१४)

It is the type of poison which exerts its effects after a time and is a combination of poisonous and non poisonous substances. Thus it doesn't affect or kill the patient immediately.

- Method of poisoning (गरविष प्रयोग):

  सौभाग्यार्थं स्त्रियः स्वेदरजोनाना अन्नगजां मलान् ।
  शत्रुप्रयुक्तांश्च गरान् प्रयच्छन्त्यन्नमिश्रितान् ।। (च.चि.२३/२३३)

The females with an intention to gain favor or attention from their male partners, mix their sweat, blood or any other excreta along with the foods and drinks. The person dreams about jackals, cat, mongoose, snake, monkey, tress and dry reservoirs.

Table 4.1 Features of Garavisha (गरविष लक्षण)

| पाण्डु | Paleness |
|---|---|
| कार्श्य | Emaciation |
| अल्प अग्नि, आध्मान | Improper digestion, abdominal distention |
| कास, श्वास, ज्वर | Cough, asthma, fever |
| अर्दित | Facial palsy |
| प्रतिलोम वायु गति | Abnormal movement of Vayu |
| अति निंद्रा | Excess sleep |
| अति चिन्ता | Excess worry |
| प्लीहोदर | Splenomegaly |
| दीन वाक् | Feeble voice |
| क्षय | Tuberculosis |
| शोफ | Oedema of different organs |
| सुश्क पाद कर | Wasting of limbs |

- ***Treatment of Garavisha*** (गरविष चिकित्सा)
    - Vamana, Pathya – ahara.
    - Suvarna Lehana to purify Hridaya. Lehana with Sharkara, Kshaudra, Tapya & Suvarna churna.
    - Churna of Murva, Amrita, Nata, Kana, Patoli, Chavya, Chitraka, Vacha, Musta & Vidanga with Takra or Ushnodaka or Mastu or Amlarasa.

- ***According to Charaka Samhita*** (च.चि.२३/१४)

Garavisha is the type of poison which is prepared artificially by the mixture of various substances. It produces diseases. Since it takes some time for this type of poison to get metabolized and to produce its toxic effects, it does not cause instantaneous death of a person. Garavisha is of 2 types; the one which is produced by the combination of non poisonous Dravya, and the other which is produced by the combination of poisonous Dravya. However, according to Acharya Kashyapa, if Visha is produced due to combination of non-poisonous Dravya, it is called Garavisha. If it is produced due to combination of poisonous Dravya, it is called Kritrima Visha.

### 4.2 Dooshivisha

Basically there are Jangama, Sthavara and Garavisha mentioned. When these Visha due to treatment gets less potent but doesn't get eliminated completely, then it causes various symptoms. This type of poison effect is called as Dooshivisha. Dooshivisha is slow poison which gradually develops over time. It is classified under Kritrima Visha by Acharaya Vagbhata.

- ***Nirukti:***

दूष + णिच् + इन् : Means anything which is impure or vitiated.

- ***Definition:***

दूषितं देशकालान्नदिवास्वप्नैरभीक्ष्णशः ।
यस्माद् दूषयते धातून् तस्माद् दूषीविषं स्मृतम् ।। (सु.क.२/३३)

On constant exposure to windy & cloudy place like Anupa Desha, rainy season, food like Kullatha, Masha, Tila and habitual day sleep. All these cause vitiation of Dhatus. This type of poison which doesn't cause any acute symptoms is called as Dooshivisha.

- ***Etiology:***

When any poison not fully eliminated from body but gets dried due to Agni, Vata or Tapa. When the potency of drug becomes less potent is called as Dooshivisha.

- ***Aggravating factors:***

  कोपं च शीतानिलदुर्दिनेषु यत्याशु, पूर्व श्रुणु तत्र रुपम्।
  (सु. क.२/२६)

This type of poison gets aggravated due to cold weather, winds, cloudy days.

- ***Purvarupa:***

  निद्रा गुरुत्वं च विजृम्भण च विश्लेषहर्षावथवा अंगमर्दः।
  (सु.क.२/३०)

Table 4.2 Purvarupa of Dooshivisha

| | |
|---|---|
| निंद्रा | Sleepiness |
| गुरुत्वं | Heaviness |
| विजृम्भणं | Yawning |
| सन्धि विश्लेष | Sense of looseness of joints |
| रोमहर्ष | Horripilation |
| अंगमर्द | Bodyache |

- ***Dooshivisha lakshana:***

  तेन् अर्दितो भिन्नपुरीषवर्णो विगन्धवैरस्यमुखः पिपासी ।
  मूर्च्छन् वमन् गद्गदवाग्विषण्णो भवेच्च दुष्योदरलिंगजुष्टः ।।
  (सु.क. २/२७)

Table 4.3 Dooshivisha lakshana

| | |
|---|---|
| भिन्न पुरीष | Diarrhoea |
| विवर्ण | Discoloration |
| वैरस्यमुख | Bad smell from mouth |
| पिपासी | Thirst |
| मूर्छा | Fainting |
| वमन | Vomiting |
| गद गद वाक् | Stammering speech |
| दूष्योदर | Various symptoms of Dushyodara. |

Table 4.4 Features according to site

| | |
|---|---|
| आमाशय | Diseases of Kapha - Vata |
| पित्ताशय | Diseases of Vata – Pitta, hair fall, loss of strength. |
| धातु | Various types of Dhatugata Vikara. |

- ***Prognosis:***

In person having good strength and which is newly manifested, it can be cured easily. A case standing more than one year is palliable. The person who is weak and has no strength, in such it is incurable.

- ***Treatment:***

1. **Shodhana:** Swedana, Vamana, Virechan.
2. **Agadapana:** Pippali, Savara, Mamsi, Dhyamaka, Paripelavam, Suvarchika, Sasuksmaila, Kanakagairik be mixed with honey. This combination is called as Vishari Agad.

**4.3 Contemporary aspects of Garavisha and Dooshivisha**

Due to our lifestyle, we are knowingly or unknowingly exposed to various types of aspects. So any harmful or less potent poison may get into our vessels of daily use and cause harms. Foods, drinks, cosmetics, toothpaste may contain poison. The alarming increase in life style disorders diseases can be attributed to these harmful daily use products.

***1. Foods:***

**Meat:** Selling meat unfit for eating, selling them as organic. Adding beef to pork sausages.

**Fish:** Selling them as wild fish even when farmed. Labelling the wrong geographic region.

**Orange juice:** Adding inferior quality juices, adding beet sugar to sweeten the natural orange juice.

**Rice:** Adding cheaper quality to basmati rice to increase the bulk and earn more profit.

**Fruits and vegetables:** Selling conventional products as organic. Labelling the wrong geographic region. Selling soya beans mixed with conventional beans without declaring it.

Table 4.5 Adulterants & its symptoms

| Food items | Adulterant | Symptoms |
|---|---|---|
| Edible oil | Argemone oil | Dropsy, glaucoma |
| Jaggery | Washing powder | Vomiting, diarrhoea |
| Tea | Colored saw dust | Cancer |
| Milk | Urea | Organ malfunction, cancer |
| Chilli powder | Brick powder | Cancer |
| Turmeric powder | Metanil yellow | Cancer |
| Wheat flour | Talcum powder | Intestinal diseases, cancer |

### *2. Drinks:*

It can be soft drink, milk, milk shakes which can be adulterated. Milk is considered as white poison owing to the presence of pesticides, insecticides, microbes, urea, excessive hormones. Heavy metals present in tea, coffee. Some colouring agents are also added to these drinks. Artificial sugar named Aspartame which is known to show carcinogenic effects. Drinking water also contains heavy metals.

### *3. Cosmetics:*

Face creams, lotions, lipsticks, sprays. Talcum powder has shown ovarian cancer effects. Imadazolidinyl present in hair dyes causes cancer. Phthalate in artificial fragrances has immune interference. Sodium Lauryl Sulphate present in oil and dirt removing creams is proven to be carcinogenic. BHA (Butylated Hydroxy Anisole) & BHT (Butylated Hydroxy Toluene) present in lipsticks and moisturizers cause harm to liver, kidney, thyroid problems.

*4. Drugs:*

Some drugs like aspirin, paracetamol, oral contraceptives have their own harmful effects. Acute overdose of aspirin can be accidental or intentional. Where as chronic over dose can be due to everyday dose built in body. Aspirin inhibits the fat metabolism which on long term use can cause Reye's syndrome. Paracetamol on chronic use can cause liver damage.

The Dooshivisha contemporary causes can be incompatible foods, agriculture pollution, environmental pollution, drugs and narcotics. These get built up in the body slowly and cause harmful effects over the time.

**Incompatible foods:** Junk foods, chicken with curd, fish with milk, hot and cold food together.

**Agriculture pollution:** Pesticides, fungicides, herbicides, rodenticides, synthetic pesticides.

**Air pollutants:** Gaseous pollutions, pesticides, carcinogens, radioactive pollutants, bioactive contaminants.

**Water pollution:** Organic pollutants, synthetic detergents, oxygen demanding wastes, toxic metals, agricultural pollutants, suspended matters.

**Soil pollution:** Plastic waste, synthetic waste, biomedical waste, E – waste, heavy metal pollution.

**Drugs:** Alcohol, steroids, quinines, tobacco, NSAIDs.

## 4.4 Role of Garavisha and Dooshivisha in the Manifestation of Diseases

- While the effect of industrialization and commercialization are widely and rapidly spreading in the society, the chances of contacts with toxins are also increasing. With the change in life style of modern civilized man.

- The risk of getting exposure to the poisons like Garavisha and Dooshivisha are also increasing day by day. There are so many sectors that can be compared to Garavisha in today's society, the prevalence of which is very high. The sectors are: Adulteration / preservatives, Cosmetics, Psychoactive drugs, Occupational poisoning.
- Now-a-days, food preservatives have a very extensive use. Many of these appear to be innocuous but there is danger in continuous use of food preserved by these agents. Carbonated cold drinks are actually a combination of phosphoric acid, sugar, caffeine, colouring agent, heavy metals and flavouring agents. Now-a-days vegetables and fruits also contain chemicals beyond permissible limits.
- In agricultural practice also the use of chemical fertilizers, pesticides pollute their growing land, poison the nearby water source and leave their residues in the food stuff.
- By taking these food products many harmful chemicals enter into the body which can cause acute, chronic or cumulative toxicity, trans-dermally causing local as well as systemic problems. Another sector in modem field i.e., occupational poisoning can also be comparable to Garavisha.
- It is occurring due to the accidental exposure to poison through skin, eyes, nose, mouth etc. As it is known that Dushivisha as such after getting inside the body immediately cannot manifest.
- Any poison (may be Sthavara, Jangama or Kritrima Visha) after exposure remain inside the body and in favourable conditions only get vitiated and manifest the symptoms. These favourable conditions include Dushita Desha, Kaala, Anna, Jatharaagni, Divaswapna, Ahitashana etc.
- In recent days already pollution has taken as an important risk factor for mankind, it includes pollution of land, air and water, the factors responsible for aggravation of Dooshivisha.

- The pollution of all these factors and use of fertilizers, chemicals, pesticides etc. in agriculture ultimately leads to the deposition of toxins in foods which in turn get into the body. Alteration of living style, food habits, exposure to different toxins etc. interfere in the digestive power of a person and due to all these factors causes harm.

**Multiple Choice Questions:**

**1.** नानाप्राण्यंगशमलविरुद्धौषधिभस्मनाम्**.... Is the shloka for?**

A. Garavisha B. Dooshivisha

C. Viruddha Ahara D. Sthavara Visha

**2.** दूषितं देशकालान्नदिवास्वप्नैरभीक्ष्णश **...... is the shloka for?**

A. Garavisha B. Dooshivisha

C. Viruddha Ahara D. Sthavara Visha

**3. Edible oil is adulterated with?**

A. Coloured saw powder B. Urea

C. Argemone oil D. Talcum powder

**4. BHA & BHT are adulterants for which substance?**

A. Drinks B. Cosmetics C. Drugs D. Foods

**5. Chilli powder is adulterated wuth?**

A. Urea B. Metanil yellow C. Brick powder D. Washing powder

**6. Reye's syndrome occurs due to long term use of which medicine?**

A. PCM B. Aspirin C. Antihistamines D. Antibiotics

**7. Which carcinogenic substance is present in hairdyes?**

A. BHA B. BHT C. Imadazolidinyl D. Sodiun Lauryl Sulphate

**8. Dropsy occurs due to adulteration in which substance?**
A. Jaggery B. Wheat flour C. Edible oil D. Milk

**9.** गद्‌गदवाग्विषण्णो भवेच्च दुष्योदरलिंगजुष्ट **..... is the Lakshana for which substance?**
A. Garavisha B. Dooshivisha
C. Viruddha Ahara D. Sthavara Visha

**10. Wheat flour is adulterated with?**
A. Metanil yellow B. Brick powder
C. Washing powder D. Talcum powder

**Answer key for MCQs:**

| | |
|---|---|
| 1 | A |
| 2 | B |
| 3 | C |
| 4 | B |
| 5 | C |

| | |
|---|---|
| 6 | B |
| 7 | C |
| 8 | C |
| 9 | B |
| 10 | D |

# Ch. 5
# Visha Upadrava & Diseases Caused Due to Exposure to Visha

## 5.1 Visha Upadrava

- विषवेगान्मदमूर्छाविषाद ह्रदयद्रवाः प्रवर्तन्ते । (च.चि.२३/४३)

मदः Intoxication
मूछाः Fainting
विषादः Depression
ह्रदयद्रवः Palpitations

ज्वरकासवमिश्वासहिध्मा तृष्णा अतिमूर्छनम् ।
विशोभेदो अतिकाठिन्यमानाहो बस्तिमूर्धरुक् ।।
श्वयथुः पूतिदंशत्वं रक्तस्त्रावो विषानिलः ।
इति षोडश निर्दिष्टा विषार्तानामुपद्रवाः ।। (अ.स.उ. ४७/२)

Table 5.1 Complications of poison, symptoms & its treatment

| Symptoms | Treatment |
|---|---|
| Jwara: Fever | Ushira, Padmaka, Ghana Kwatha + sugar + honey. |
| Kasa: Cough | Bharangi, Utpala, Kesara, Ajaji with Tandula. |
| Shwasa: Dyspnoea | Draksha, Nagara, Krishna, Vara, Ghana added with ghee + honey. |
| Vami: Vomiting | Kwatha of Bilwamula added with Maricha. |
| Hikka: Hiccups | Powder of Shanka, Kanaka, Swarna Gairika. |
| Trushna: Thirst | Drink Laja Tarpana with sugar. Apply body organs with Chandana paste. |
| Murchha: Fainting | Cover the head with milk ghee, cool sugarcane juice. |
| Atisara: Diarrhoea | Nagara with curds. Lodhra, Mocharasa, Dhataki + Tandula. |
| Vibandha: Constipation | Triphala with warm water internally. |

| Anaha: Flatulence | Kvatha of Triphala, Aragwadha, Vyaghri. |
|---|---|
| Bastishula: Bladder pain | Introduce Phalavarti. Haritaki + Trivritta + ghee. |
| Shirashula: Headache | Kakoli, Draksha, Sharkara with cold water Nasya. |
| Shvayathu: Swelling | Milk boiled with Kustuka, Devdaru. Goat milk boiled with Pippali. |
| Putidamsha: Bad smell | Paste of leaf buds of Madhuka, Tila, Saindhava, Abhaya + leaves of Nimba. |
| Raktasrava: Bleeding disorder | Coat the wound with Darvi. Ghee processed with Maricha and sugar. Nasya with Sitopala, honey, ghee, goat's milk. |
| Vishavata: Vata aggravated due to poison | Ghee made of Pippali, Bhallataka, Bilva be drank. Eranda Taila mixed with goat meat juice. Ghee + oil + goat meat juice. |

## 5.2 Drug induced toxicity

The adverse effects of drugs caused by its use in therapeutic or non – therapeutic doses.

- **Causes:** It can be caused due to over – ingestion of medicine. The threshold dose in some person can be over dose in the other. When dose crosses the prescribed amount or the prescribed dose is high causes drug induced toxicity. It can also occur as an adverse drug reaction, where the normal therapeutic dose of the drug causes unwanted, harmful yet unintentional side effects. The toxicity and its severity depends on:

a) Chemical structure.
b) How much drug can be absorbed.
c) The body's capacity to detoxify and eliminate the substance.

- **Symptoms of drug toxicity:** Diarrhoea, nausea, dizziness, stomachache, vomiting, weakness. In more severe cases it can be Ataxia, muscle twitches, tremors, nystagmus, seizures, slurred speech. Carbamazapine, often used to treat schizophrenia causes blurred vision, dizziness, nystagmus, trouble walking and altered levels of consciousness.

- **Diagnosis:** Assay of electrolytes with anion gap calculation, complete blood count, coagulation studies, arterial blood gas, creatinine & transaminase levels.

- **Treatment:** If the toxicity results from an acute overdose, a person may undergo stomach pumping to remove drugs that have not yet been absorbed. Activated charcoal is another drug toxicity treatment option. It can be used to bind the drug, preventing it from being absorbed into the blood. If this approach is used, the drug is eliminated from the body through stool. Other medications may also be given as an antidote for drug toxicity.

### 5.3 Occupational Hazards

Any hazard which is associated with a specific industry or occupation is called as Occupational hazard. Any physical, chemical, biological or psychological factors present in work place can cause occupational hazards.

- Types of occupational hazards:

*A.* ***Safety:*** Conditions, substance or objects which can harm workers like working from height, spills on the floor, machinery with moving parts, confined spaces, exposed electrical wirings, steep steps.

***B. Biological:*** In farms, zoo, veterinary clinics there can be exposure to molds, fungi, blood, animal droppings and insect bites.

***C. Chemical:*** Many products like environmental smokes, cleaning products, acids, pesticides, carbon monoxide, inflammable liquids.

- **Inhalation** – that is breathing in toxic vapours or small chemical particles

- **Absorption** – such as direct exposure to the skin by touching a chemical substance without any protection such as wearing gloves.
- **Injection** – that is when a sharp contaminated object or needle accidentally penetrates a worker's body (such as hand or foot)
- **Ingestion** – that is when toxins are accidentally swallowed.
- **Chemical asphyxiants** deprive the body of oxygen; interrupting the transfer and use of oxygen by the bloodstream. Eg: Carbon monoxide.
- **Chemical corrosives** cause visible and/or irreversible changes to the composition of a material due to direct contact. Similarly, these can also cause a localized reaction in the human body at the point of contact. Eg: Sulphuric acid.
- **Chemical hazards** that are classified as irritants cause harm to the eyes, skin, or respiratory tract of a person. Irritants are either highly, moderately, or slightly water-soluble. The hazards can manifest as redness, rashes, inflammation, coughing, or haemorrhaging. Irritants are mostly short-term severe illnesses but can also have long-lasting side effects in some people. Eg: Nickel acid.
- **Carcinogens** are cancer-causing chemical substances, and a small amount of such a chemical is enough to severely harm human health. The hazards of such chemical substances will only appear many years after exposure. There are over 200 known human carcinogens. Eg: Benzene.

***D. Physical:*** These can harm without actually touching the body. Extreme low and high temperatures, radiations, direct sunlight.

- **Vibrations:** There are risks connected to working with vibrating equipment and plant which need to be assessed and managed. Evidence also shows that people who experience vibration and noise at the same time are more likely to suffer hearing loss and musculoskeletal problems, than people exposed to noise or vibration alone.

- **Noise**: Excessive noise is considered when voice needs to be raised for a person standing 1m away. Excessive noise can lead to hearing loss (temporary or permanent), tinnitus, affects psychological health leading to anxiety, depression, fatigue and sleeplessness.
- **Body stressing**: Loss of grip strength, loss of mobility, feeling tension in muscles, incomplete tasks due to repeated fatigue.
- **Confined spaces**: These are smaller areas not made to work on regular basis. When work done in these areas leads to improper ventilation, airborne diseases and suffocation due to increased CO2 levels.
- **Heat**: Occurs in professions like commercial kitchens, laundries, factories where there is improper heat removal form the rooms. Environmental conditions (such as air temperature, humidity, sunlight, and air speed), especially on sequential days. Presence of heat sources (e.g., hot tar ovens or furnaces) in the work area.

***E. Work place organization hazards:*** Violence, lack of respect, discrimination, sexual harassment or any behavior which is harmful for physical and psychological health.

***F. Ergonomic:*** Initially these cause short term problems like sore muscles but on continuing the same activity can lead to major health damages.

The steps to deal with work place hazards are:

- **Anticipation & recognition**: Doing prior preparation and identifying any hazard s and possibility of any worker being affected by it.
- **Assess**: If there is possibility of hazard then it must be assessed for its potential to cause harm.
- **Control**: If the hazard is identified then all steps necessary to control it should be taken.

- **Evaluation**: Assess if the control is effective and whether the hazards are controlled effectively or not.
- **Substitution**: Use of less harmful materials, change in process equipment or change of process.
- **Engineering controls**: Isolation within a containment structure, Ventilation with local exhaust and general exhaust, job rotation schedules, work rest cycles.
- **Hygiene facilities & practice**: Washing hands after touching materials and before having food, avoid touching eyes, nose, lips with contaminated hands, avoid drinking or smoking in work places.
- **Protective equipment**: Respirators, hearing protectors, safety clothing and protective clothing.

This comes as the duty of employers under:

- **OHSA (Occupation Health and Safety Act)** section 25(2)(h).
- Section 3 of **Control of Exposure to Biological or Chemical Agents, Regulation 833.**
- Section 5.1, 5.2, 5.3 of Regulation 833 **Mines and Mining Plants, Regulation 854.**

- **Silicosis:** The occupational hazard disease caused due inhaling minute particles of silica leading to swelling and scarring. Occurs in people working at mining, stone making, ceramics, pottery, demolition & construction.

  ***Types:***

  **Acute** occurs on extreme exposure made of large particles for several months.

  **Sub-acute** occurs over a period of 2 – 5 years.

  **Chronic** occurs over 10 years period when there is exposure to breathable dusts.

**Symptoms**: Persistent coughing, coughing out sputum, shortness of breath, fatigue, weakness, inflammation with fibrosis of lungs.

**Diagnosis**: X-ray, CT-scan, Pulmonary Function Test, Broncho-alveolar lavage, Monteux test, lung biopsy.

**Treatment**: Use personal protective equipment, wear mask during work, avoid smoking and drinking, use bronchodilators to improve air flow, get pneumococcal vaccines.

- **Asbestosis**: The lung disease caused due to inhalation of asbestos fibers. There occurs hardening of lungs due to fibrosis making breathing difficult.

  **Symptoms:** The symptoms vary upon the severity. It may also take 10 – 15 years after the exposure. The early symptom may be shortness of breaths. Chest pain, chest tightness, clubbing of nails, coughing, crackling sound on inhalation, fatigue, trouble on exertional work.

  **Complications**: Lung cancer, mesothelioma, right sided heart failure, respiratory failure.

  **Diagnosis**: X-ray, CT-scan, Pulmonary Function Test, Spirometry, Bronchoscopy.

  **Treatment**: Oxygen therapy, pulmonary rehabilitation by exercises and behavioral therapy, lung transplant surgery, anti-fibrotics medicine which slows down the scarring from worsening. Active and passive smoking be quit. Hand wash hygiene be maintained. Nutritious foods be intaken and exercise like brisk walking should be done.

- **Anthracosis:** Long term inhalation and deposition of coal dust on lungs is called as Anthracosis. It is also called as Black Lung Disease. Inhaled coal dust progressively builds up in the lungs and leads to inflammation, fibrosis, and in worse cases, necrosis.

**Types**: Anthracosis, Simple coal worker's pneumoconiosis, Progressive massive fibrosis.

**Symptoms**: Cough with or without black sputum, shortness of breaths, chest tightness, clubbing of nails.

**Diagnosis**: X-ray, CT-scan, Pulmonary Function Test, Spirometry, Bronchoscopy.

**Treatment:** Oxygen therapy, pulmonary rehabilitation by exercises and behavioral therapy, lung transplant surgery, anti-fibrotics medicine which slows down the scarring from worsening. Active and passive smoking be quit.

- **Byssinosis**: Byssinosis is a rare lung disease. It's caused by inhaling hemp, flax, and cotton particles and is sometimes referred to as brown lung disease. Occurs almost exclusively in people who work with unprocessed cotton. People who open bales of cotton during the first stage of processing are at the highest risk.

  **Symptoms**: The symptoms show increase during work week and improved at weekends. Usually starts with shortness of breaths, tightness of chest, wheezing and coughing. Fever, muscle pain, joint pain, shivering, tiredness, dry coughing. The symptoms decrease when there is decrease in exposure to dust.

  **Diagnosis**: X-ray, CT-scan, Pulmonary Function Test, Spirometry, Bronchoscopy.

  **Treatment**: Oxygen therapy, pulmonary rehabilitation by exercises and behavioral therapy, lung transplant surgery, anti-fibrotics medicine which slows down the scarring from worsening. Active and passive smoking be quit.

## 5.4 Allergic Manifestation

Allergic reactions occur when immune system reacts to pollens, bee venom, pet dander, foods that usually doesn't cause any reaction in other people. The allergic reaction may occur from minor irritations to anaphylaxis.

Table 5.2 Factors for allergic manifestation & its symptoms

| **Factors** | **Symptoms** |
|---|---|
| Foods | Pain in abdomen, diarrhoea, indigestion, nausea, tingling lips, hives, rashes. |
| Inhalants | Runny nose, congestion, itchy eyes, nose, throat, sneezing, loss of smell, rashes. |
| Pets | Congestion, runny nose, sneezing, puffy eyes, watery eyes, coughing, itching, skin rash. |
| Mold | Runny nose, post nasal drip, sneezing, shortness of breath, throat irritation. |
| Pollen | Wheezing, sneezing, runny nose, nasal congestion, shortness of breath, chest tightness. |
| Latex | Blisters, rashes, redness, runny nose, sneezing, throat irritation, watery eyes. People with latex allergy also may avoid peaches, tomatoes, kiwi, peanuts, chestnuts, figs. |
| Insect | Hives, itching and swelling in areas other than the sting site. Abdominal cramping, vomiting, intense nausea or diarrhoea, tightness in the chest and difficulty in breathing, hoarseness of voice or swelling of the tongue or throat, difficulty swallowing. |
| Atopic dermatitis | Itching, redness, flaky skin. |

- **Anaphylaxis:** It is a severe life threatening reaction occurring after seconds or minutes after the exposure to allergic substances. The immune system releases amounts of chemicals that causes the reaction.

  **Causes:** Cow's milk, soy, peanuts, shellfish, wheat, treenuts, seeds, eggs.

  **Symptoms**: Swelling in lips, throat and tongue. Shortness of breath, hives, difficulty in swallowing, rashes, abdominal pain, cramps, diarrhoea, vomiting, wheezing.

  **Life threatening symptoms**: Lightheaded feeling, drop in blood pressure, increased heart rates, sudden weakness, cardiac arrest, unconsciousness.

**Stages of anaphylaxis:**

**Stage 1**: Mild anaphylaxis is the first stage and can cause symptoms like skin rash or redness, itching or hives.

**Stage 2**: Moderate anaphylaxis happens when there are more widespread and extensive symptoms like skin rash and hives that are spreading or mild swelling in their lips or tongue.

**Stage 3**: Severe anaphylaxis happens next. There are signs of difficulty breathing, extensive swelling, weak pulse or dizziness. A person in stage three anaphylaxis is experiencing a condition called anaphylactic shock.

**Stage 4**: Life-threatening anaphylaxis is the last stage and there occurs losing consciousness, being unable to breathe and having inadequate blood flow to vital organs and there is need for immediate treatment.

**Treatment**: Lay the person supine and if there is breathing problem sitting position makes breathing easier. If person is unconscious, lift the chin to open airway. Intubation be done. Perform tracheostomy. IV fluids with medication help strengthen the heart and circulatory system. IV fluids, antihistamines, steroids be given when the person becomes stable.

### 5.5 Endocrine Disruptors

The endocrine system is a network of glands that produce hormones useful for the body.

Endocrine disruptors are the chemicals that interfere with the normal functions. These are called as Endocrine Disrupting Chemicals. Endocrine disruptors affect the body in 3 ways:

1. Block the pathway between natural hormones and its receptors.
2. Directly affecting the gland causing it to produce too much or too less hormone.
3. They mimic a hormone, causing body to overreact or to react at the wrong time.

**Sources of endocrine disruptors:** Industrial, Agriculture, Residential.

**Brominated flame retardants (BFRs)** are used in electronics, clothing, and furniture such as sofas and mattresses to reduce flammability. Unfortunately, these chemicals also have been linked to abnormal hormone function in the thyroid, which plays a critical role in foetal and childhood development.

**Polychlorinated biphenyls (PCBs)** were used in hundreds of industrial and commercial applications due to their non-flammability, as well as chemical stability and insulating properties. Although the EPA banned their manufacture in the United States in 1979, PCBs are still present in insulation, electrical equipment, caulking, oil-based paint.

**Phthalates** interfere with the production of androgen

(testosterone), a hormone critical in male development and relevant to females as well. Phthalates are used in hundreds of products, including many food and beverage containers and plastic wraps. Plastic containers, which contain phthalates, have the number "3" and “V” or “PVC” in the recycling symbol.

**Bisphenol A (BPA)** is one of the best known and most pervasive. In humans, it is linked to reduced egg quality and other aspects of egg viability in patients seeking fertility treatment.

**Chlorpyrifos**, an insecticide used in commercial agriculture, is a potent neurotoxicant that causes developmental delays, attention problems, and ADHD in children. It accumulates in soil, water, food, and air, as well as in buildings.

**DDT** might be associated with breast cancer, preterm birth, early pregnancy loss, reduced semen quality, disrupted menstruation, and problems with lactation.

**Dioxins** are present in manufacturing substances and spread when burn.

**Perfluoroalkyl**.

**Multiple Choice Questions:**

**1. Kwatha of Aragwadha, Triphala, Vyaghri is drank for which Visha Upadrava?**

A. Jwara B. Shwasa C. Anaha D. Vami

**2. Which substance is a chemical corrosive?**

A. Sulphuric acid B. Carbon monoxide

C. Benzene D. Nickel acid

**3. विषवेगान्मदमूर्छाविषाद हृदयद्रवाः प्रवर्तन्ते........ shloka for Visha Upadrava is from which sthana of Charak Smahita?**

A. Kalpasthana B. Nidanasthana
C. Chikita sthana D. Siddhi sthana

**4. Which of the following is a physical occupational hazard?**
A. Inhalation B. Confined spaces C. Ingestion D. Absorption

**5. Which of the following is chemical occupational hazard?**
A. Carcinogen B. Vibrations C. Heat D. Body stressing

**6. Mesothalamia is a complication of which occupational disease?**
A. Silicosis B. Anthracosis C. Asbestosis D. Byssinosis

**7. Allergy of peaches, kiwis, tomatoes can also be found in people with allergies of?**
A. Inhalants B. Mold C. Pollen D. Latex

**8. Which of the following is a potent neurotoxin?**
A. Pthalates B. Chlorpyrifos C.PCB D. BFR

**9. Abnormal thyroid hormone function is related to which of the following?**
A. DDT B. Dioxins C. BFR D. BPA

**10. Which of the following interferes with testosterone production?**
A. Pthalates B. DDT C. BPA D. PCB

**Answer key for MCQs:**

| | |
|---|---|
| 1 | C |
| 2 | A |
| 3 | C |
| 4 | B |
| 5 | A |

| | |
|---|---|
| 6 | C |
| 7 | D |
| 8 | B |
| 9 | C |
| 10 | A |

# Ch. 6
# Environmental Toxicology

## 6.1 Vishakta Vayu, Jala, Bhumi (Air, water and land pollution)

Environment includes the surroundings or conditions in which a person, animal or plant operates, including air, water, land, natural resources, flora, fauna, humans and their interrelation.

- **Toxicity:** Toxicity refers to the potential of a substance to produce an adverse or harmful effect on a living organism. A toxicant is an agent that can produce an adverse effect in a biological system, seriously damaging its structure or function or causing death.
- **Toxins:** Metals, therapeutic drugs, industrial chemicals, pollutants, pesticides, fuels, herbicides and abused drugs (exogenous). Bacterial toxins, parasitic products, bile, hormones (endogenous). Environmental toxins are cancer-causing chemicals and endocrine disruptors, both human-made and naturally occurring, that can harm our health by disrupting sensitive biological systems.
- Environmental Toxicity: Environmental Toxicology is a multidisciplinary field of science concerned with the study of harmful effects of various chemical, biological and physical agents on living organisms. There are many sources of environmental toxicity that can lead to the presence of toxicants in our food, water and air. Pollutants are the prime source for environmental toxicity.

**Pollution:** Pollution may be defined as an addition of undesirable material into the environment as a result of human activities.

A **pollutant** may be defined as a physical, chemical or biological substance, released into the environment which is directly or indirectly harmful to human and other living organisms.

- **Vishakta Vayu Lakshana and chikitsa:**

धूमेअनिले वा विषसम्प्रयुक्ते खगाः श्रमार्ताः प्रपतन्ति भूमौ।
कासप्रतिश्यायशिरोरुजश्च भवन्तितीव्रा नयनामायाश्च।।
लाक्षाहरिद्रातिविषाभयाब्दहरेणुकैलादलवक्रकुष्ठम्।
प्रियङ्गुकां चाप्यनले निधाय धूमानिलौ चापि विशोधयेत।।
(सु.क. ३/१६–१७)

If the air is poisoned than it causes birds to fall on ground being exhausted. Develops severe coughing, nasal catarrh, headache and severe eye diseases.

**Treatment**: Laksha, Haridra, Ativisha, Abhaya, Musta, Harenuka, Eladala, Tagara, Priyangu, Kushtha be put on fire and the smoke formed purifies the air.

- **Air pollution:**
    - A major source of air pollution results from the burning of fossil fuels. Vehicle and factory emissions are common sources of this type of air pollution.
    - The burning of fossil fuels contributes to the formation of smog, a dense layer of particulate matter that hangs like a cloud over many major cities and industrial zones.
    - Air pollution contributes to respiratory problems such as asthma, lung cancer, chronic bronchitis, and other lung ailments.
    - Nitrogen and sulphur oxides in the air contribute to acid rain, which is a form of precipitation with a lower

(more acidic) pH than normal.

- Acid rain harms forests, species that live in water bodies, and degrades outdoor statues, monuments, and buildings.

**Types of Air Pollutants**: There are two types of air pollutants:

**Primary Pollutants**: The pollutants that directly cause air pollution are known as primary pollutants. Sulphur-dioxide emitted from factories is a primary pollutant.

**Secondary Pollutants**: The pollutants formed by the intermingling and reaction of primary pollutants are known as secondary pollutants. Smog, formed by the intermingling of smoke and fog, is a secondary pollutant.

***Air pollution control measures include:***

1. By minimising and reducing the use of fire and fire products.
2. Since industrial emissions are one of the major causes of air pollution, the pollutants can be controlled or treated at the source itself to reduce its effects. For example, if the reactions of a certain raw material yield a pollutant, then the raw materials can be substituted with other less polluting materials.
3. Fuel substitution is another way of controlling air pollution. In many parts of India, petrol and diesel are being replaced by CNG – Compressed Natural Gas fueled vehicles. These are mostly adopted by vehicles that aren't fully operating with ideal emission engines.
4. Although there are many practices in India, which focus on repairing the quality of air, most of them are either forgotten or not being enforced properly. There are still a lot of vehicles on roads which haven't been tested for vehicle emissions.
5. Another way of controlling air pollution caused by industries is to modify and maintain existing pieces of equipment so that

the emission of pollutants is minimised.

6. Sometimes controlling pollutants at the source is not possible. In that case, we can have process control equipment to control the pollution.
7. A very effective way of controlling air pollution is by diluting the air pollutants.
8. The last and the best way of reducing the ill effects of air pollution is tree plantation. Plants and trees reduce a large number of pollutants in the air. Ideally, planting trees in areas of high pollution levels will be extremely effective.

- **Vishakta Jala Lakshana and Chikitsa:**

दुष्टम् जलम् पिच्छिलमुग्रगंधि फेनान्वितं राजिभिरावृतं च।
मण्डूकमत्स्यम् म्रियते विहङ्गा मत्ताश्च सानूपचराभ्रमन्ति।।
मज्जन्ति ये चात्रनराश्चनागास्ते छर्दिमोहज्वरदाहशोफान्।
ऋ(ग)च्छन्ति तेषामपहृत्य दोषान् दुष्टम् जलं शोधयितुं यतेत।।
(सु.क. ३/७–८)

Poisoned water is Slimy, bad smelling, frothy, lines on the surface, frogs and fishes can't survive. On immersing in this water vomiting, fever, delusion, burning sensation occurs.

**Treatment:**

धवाश्वकर्णासनपारिभद्रान् सपाटलान् सिद्धकमोक्षकौ च।
दग्ध्वा सराजद्रुमसोमवल्कांस्तभ्दस्म शीतं वितरेत् सरःसु।।
भस्माञ्जलिं चापि घटे निधाय विशोधयेदीप्सितमेवमम्भः।
(सु क९–१०)

Dhava, Ashwakarna, Paribhadra, Asana, Patala, Mokshaka, Siddhaka, Rajadruma, Somavalkal be burnt on fire and ash be spread on water bodies and put in pots of drinking water and when needed.

**Water pollution**

- A major source of water pollution is runoff from agricultural fields, industrial sites, or urban areas.
- Runoff disrupts the water body's natural balance. For example, agricultural runoff typically includes fertilizer or toxic chemicals.
- Fertilizer can cause algal blooms (an explosive growth of algae), choking out other plants and decreasing the amount of available oxygen necessary for the survival of other species.
- Raw sewage is another type of water pollutant. When sewage gets into the drinking water supply, serious stomach and digestive issues may result, including the spread of diseases such as typhoid or dysentery.
- A third source of water pollution is trash. Improperly disposed of items, such as plastic bags, fishing line, and other materials may accumulate in the water and lead to the premature death of animals that get tangled within the garbage.
- The effect of water pollution depends upon the type of pollutants and their concentration. Also, the location of water bodies is an important factor to determine the levels of pollution.
- Water bodies in the vicinity of urban areas are extremely polluted. This is the result of dumping garbage and toxic chemicals by industrial and commercial establishments.
- Water pollution drastically affects aquatic life. It affects their metabolism, and behaviour, and causes illness and eventual death. Dioxin is a chemical that causes a lot of problems from reproduction to uncontrolled cell growth or cancer. This chemical is bio accumulated in fish, chicken and meat. Chemicals such as this travel up the food chain before entering the human body.
- The effect of water pollution can have a huge impact on the food chain. It disrupts the food chain. Cadmium and lead are some toxic substances, these pollutants upon entering the

food chain through animals (fish when consumed by animals, humans) can continue to disrupt at higher levels.

- Minimata incident: In 1932, a factory in Minamata City, Japan began dumping its industrial effluent – Methylmercury, into the surrounding bay and the sea. Methylmercury is incredibly toxic to humans and animals alike, causing a wide range of neurological disorders.

**Water pollution control measures include:**

1. Rather than releasing sewage waste into water bodies, it is better to treat them before discharge.
2. Practising this can reduce the initial toxicity and the remaining substances can be degraded and rendered harmless by the water body itself.
3. If the secondary treatment of water has been carried out, then this can be reused in sanitary systems and agricultural fields.
4. A very special plant, the Water Hyacinth can absorb dissolved toxic chemicals such as cadmium and other such elements. Establishing these in regions prone to such kinds of pollutants will reduce the adverse effects to a large extent.
5. Some chemical methods that help in the control of water pollution are precipitation, the ion exchange process, reverse osmosis, and coagulation.

- **Vishakta Bhumi Lakshana and chikitsa:**

क्षितिप्रदेशम् विषदूषीतं तु शिलातलं तीर्थमथेरिणम् वा।।
स्पृशन्ति गात्रेण तु येन येन गोवाजिनागोष्ट्रखरा नरा वा।
तच्छूनतां यात्यथ दह्यते च विशीर्यते रोमनखं तथैव।।
तत्राप्यनन्तां सह सर्वागन्धैः पिष्ट्वा सुराभिर्विनियोज्य मार्गम्।
सिन्चेत् पयोभिः सुमृदन्वतैस्तं विडङ्गपाठाकटभीजलैर्वा।।
(सु क / १०–१२)

When poisoned sand dunes or land touches the organs of cows, buffalo, elephant, camel, men causes burning. There occurs hair fall and nails fall. There occurs oedema.

**Treatment:** Durva + Ela, Karpura dissolved in honey or jaggery be mixed with Sura and made into paste. And should be sprinkled on poisoned areas. Water boiled with Vidanga, Patha, Katabhi should be sprinkled.

**Land pollution:**

- Soil pollution is a form of land pollution in which the soil's upper layer is harmed.
- Overuse of chemical fertilizers, soil degradation caused by running water, and other pest control measures contribute to the loss of agricultural land, forest cover, and grazing pastures, among other things.
- Soil can become polluted by industrial sources or the improper disposal of toxic chemical substances. Common sources of soil pollution include asbestos, lead, PCBs, and overuse of pesticides or herbicides.
- Additionally, various compounds get into the soil from the atmosphere, for instance with precipitation water, as well as by wind activity or other types of soil disturbances, and from surface water bodies and shallow groundwater flowing through the soil.
- Humans can be affected by soil pollution through the inhalation of gases emitted from soils moving upward, or through the inhalation of matter that is disturbed and transported by the wind because of the various human activities on the ground.
- Soil pollution may cause a variety of health problems, starting with headaches, nausea, fatigue, skin rash, eye irritation and potentially resulting in more serious conditions like neuromuscular blockage, kidney and liver damage and various forms of cancer.

**Effects of Land Pollution are:**

- **Climate Change** – Land contamination, such as that caused by mining, farming, and factories, may allow harmful chemicals to enter the soil and water. These chemicals have the potential to kill animals and plants, destroying the food chain. Landfills emit methane, a greenhouse gas that contributes to global warming.
- **Acid Rain** – Forests, especially those at higher elevations, are also harmed by acid rain and fog. Acid deposits deplete vital nutrients like calcium and allow aluminum to be released into the soil, making it difficult for trees to absorb water. Acids also damage the leaves and needles of trees.
- **Deterioration of fields** – A chain reaction occurs as a result of soil contamination. It alters soil biodiversity, decreases soil organic matter, and reduces soil's filtering ability. It also contaminates water contained in the soil and groundwater, resulting in nutrient imbalances in the soil.
- **Respiratory health problems** – Air pollution can irritate your airways, causing shortness of breath, coughing, wheezing, asthma attacks, and chest pain. Lung cancer, heart attacks, strokes, and, in the worst-case scenario, premature death are all risks associated with air pollution exposure.

**Land pollution control measures are:**

- To reduce land emissions, reduce, reuse, and recycle. It is essential to practice reforestation and afforestation. Organic fertilizers, an integrated pest control method, and crop rotation can all be used by farmers.
- One of the most important ways to help minimize landfill waste, protect natural resources, preserve wildlife, reduce noise, reduce energy use, and slow global warming is to incorporate recycling habits into your everyday life.
- Reforestation avoids river and lake silting by reducing

surface erosion and preserving the fertile topsoil. It prevents the soil surface from sealing and cuts down on the amount of rainwater that runs off.

- When compared to petroleum-based plastics, biodegradable plastics produce significantly less waste. As biodegradable plastics degrade, they decompose into nontoxic, harmless components.

## 6.2 Effects of Biological, Chemical and Nuclear Warfare

- Biological warfare:

Biological weapons have been used in a few instances in the past by terrorist organizations.

**Year 1155:** Emperor Barbarossa poisons water wells with human bodies, Tortona Italy.

**Year 1346:** Mongols catapult the bodies of plague victims over the city walls of Caffa, Crimean peninsula.

**Year 1495:** Spanish mix wine with blood of leprosy patients to sell to their French foes, Naples, Italy.

**Year 1650:** Polish fire saliva from rabies dogs towards their enemies.

**Year 1675:** First deal between German and French forces not to use poisonous bullets.

**Year 1763:** British distribute blankets from smallpox patients to native Americans.

**Year 1797:** Napoleon floods the plains around Mantua, Italy to enhance the spread of malaria.

**Year 1863:** Confederates sell clothing from yellow fever and smallpox to union troops, USA.

- **Anthrax** caused by Bacillus anthracis abused 1st World war,

2nd World war, Soviet Union 1979, Japan 1995.

- **Haemorrhagic fever** caused by Marburg virus, Ebola virus, Arena virus abused Soviet bioweapons program.
- **Plague** caused by Yersinia pestis abused in 14th century Europe and 2nd World war.
- **Smallpox** caused by Variola major abused in 18th century North America.
- **Tularemia** caused by Francisella tularensis abused in 2nd World war.
- **Cholera** caused by Vibrio cholerae used in 2nd World war.
- **Encephalitis** caused by Alpha virus in 2nd World war.
- **Food poisoning** caused by Salmonella, Shigella in 2nd World war.
- **Glanders** caused by Burkholderia mallei used in 1st World war.
- Biological agents were extensively used in many parts of Africa from the sixteenth century AD, most of the time in the form of poisoned arrows, or powder spread on the war front as well as poisoning of horses and water supply of the enemy forces.
- In Borgu, there were specific mixtures to kill, hypnotize, make the enemy bold, and to act as an antidote against the poison of the enemy as well.
- Biological weapons are difficult to detect, economical and easy to use, making them appealing to terrorists. The cost of a biological weapon is estimated to be about 0.05 percent the cost of a conventional weapon in order to produce similar numbers of mass casualties per kilometre square.
- Moreover, their production is very easy as common technology can be used to produce biological warfare agents, like that used in production of vaccines, foods, spray devices, beverages and antibiotics.
- Entomological warfare (EW) is a type of biological warfare that uses insects to attack the enemy. The concept has existed

for centuries and research and development have continued into the modern era.

- EW has been used in battle by Japan and several other nations have developed and been accused of using an entomological warfare program. EW may employ insects in a direct attack or as vectors to deliver a biological agent, such as plague.
- Essentially, EW exists in three varieties. One type of EW involves infecting insects with a pathogen. The insects then act as a vector infecting any person or animal they might bite.
- Another type of EW is a direct insect attack against crops; the insect may not be infected with any pathogen but instead represents a threat to agriculture.
- The final method uses uninfected insects, such as bees or wasps, to directly attack the enemy.
- Synthetic biology could be used in the future to design novel types of biological warfare agents:

1. Would demonstrate how to render a vaccine ineffective.
2. Would confer resistance to therapeutically useful antibiotics or antiviral agents.
3. Would enhance the virulence of a pathogen or render a non-pathogenic virulent.
4. Would increase the transmissibility of a pathogen.
5. Would alter the host range of a pathogen.
6. Would enable the evasion of diagnostic/detection tools.
7. Would enable the weaponization of a biological agent or toxin.

**Chemical Warfare:**

- Chemical warfare (CW) is defined as warfare that involves using of toxic properties of chemical substances as weapons or ammunitions.
- Use of toxins such as ricine, botulinum toxin, etc. fall under this category.
- Nearly seventy different chemicals are marked as weapons

for chemical warfare.

- Among the Weapons of Mass Destruction (WMD), chemical warfare is probably one of the most brutal created by mankind. CW agents are extremely toxic synthetic chemicals that can be dispersed as a gas, liquid or aerosol or as agents adsorbed to particles to become a powder.
- Ethyl bromoacetate and chloroacetone were used as chemical weapons during the First World War.
- In modern warfare, chemical weapons were first used in World war 1 (1914–18).
- In the years since then, chemical arms have been employed numerous times, most notably in the Iran – Iraq War (1980–88) and the Syrian Civil War and the Soviet Union (1945–91), built up enormous stockpiles of chemical weapons.
- Not all poisonous substances are considered suitable for weaponization, or use as chemical weapons.
- Thousands of such chemical compounds exist, but only a few dozen have been used as chemical warfare agents since 1900.
- The compounds of most utility must be highly toxic but not too difficult to handle. Furthermore, the chemical must be able to withstand the heat developed when delivered in a bursting shell, bomb, mine, or warhead.
- Finally, it must be resistant to water and oxygen in the atmosphere in order to be effective when dispersed.

**Types of chemical agents:**

- Choking agents: Chlorine, phosgene, diphosgene, chloropicrin, ethyldichlorasine, perfluoroisoboxylene. Gas mask and other protective equipment were used against these agents.
- Blister agents: Sulphur mustard, nitrogen mustard, phosgene oxime, phenyldichlorarsine, and lewisite. Delivered in liquid or vapour form, such weapons burn the skin, eyes, windpipe, and lungs. Protection against blister agents requires an effective gas mask and protective over-garments.

- Blood agents: Hydrogen-Cyanide or Cyanogen chloride. When inhaled, these agents prevent the transfer of oxygen to the cells, causing the body to asphyxiate. The best defence against blood agents is an effective gas mask.
- The most lethal and important chemical weapons contain nerve agents. G-series agents, or G agents, include GA (tabun), GB (sarin), GD (soman), and GF (cyclosarin).
- Tear gas and vomiting agents have been produced to control riots and unruly crowds. Commonly used tear gases are chloracetophenone, chloropicrin.
- Herbicides can be used to destroy enemy crops and foliage cover. Eg: Agent Orange.

**Defence against chemical weapons:**

1. Chemical detectors have been developed to help identify levels and places of contamination.
2. These include chemically treated litmus paper used to determine the presence of chemical agents. Other sensors may include handheld assays, vehicles equipped with scoops and laboratory analysis tools, and both point and standoff sensors.
3. Automatic field alarm systems are employed by some military forces to alert personnel to the presence of chemical agents.
4. Well-equipped troops are supplied with hypodermic needles filled with antidotes to be administered in the event of toxic poisoning from nerve agents. For example, atropine shots can be injected to fight the effects of nerve gas exposures.

**Nuclear warfare:**

- The device designed to release energy in an explosive, nuclear fusion, or a combination of the two processes. Fission weapons are commonly referred to as atomic bombs. Fusion weapons are also referred to as hydrogen bombs.
- The atomic bomb dropped on Hiroshima, Japan, in 1945, containing only about 64 kg (140 pounds) of highly enriched

Uranium, released energy equalling about 15 kilotons of chemical explosive.

- That blast immediately produced a strong shock wave, enormous amounts of heat, and lethal ionizing radiation.
- Convection currents created by the explosion drew dust and other debris into the air, creating the mushroom-shaped cloud that has since become the virtual signature of a nuclear explosion.
- In addition, radioactive debris was carried by winds high into the atmosphere, later to settle to Earth as radioactive fallout.
- The enormous toll in destruction, death, injury, and sickness produced by the explosions at Hiroshima.
- The first nuclear weapons were bombs delivered by aircraft. Later, warheads were developed for strategic ballistic missiles, which have become by far the most important nuclear weapons.
- **Radiation poisoning**, also called "**radiation sickness**" or a "**creeping dose**", is a form of damage to organ tissue due to excessive exposure to ionizing radiation.
- Lethal radiation syndromes, include prodromal syndrome, bone marrow death.
- CNS death: vomiting, nausea, diarrhoea, drowsiness, lethargy, tremors, delirium, seizures, heat prostration, coma, respiratory failure, death.
- Gastrointestinal death: gastric pain, anorexia, nausea, vomiting, diarrhoea.

**Short term effects:**

- Erythema lasting for more than 10 days.
- Lungs: inflammation, loss of epithelial cells, oedema, occlusion of airway, fibrosis.
- Ovaries: suppression of menstruation or permanent sterility.
- Testicles: low sperm count, loss of libido or permanent sterility.

**Long term effects:**

- Cataract induction, cancer induction, peri-natal mortality, severe mental sub normality.
- Infectious diseases: dysentery, typhoid, salmonellosis, cholera, infectious hepatitis, meningococcal meningitis, tuberculosis, diphtheria, whooping cough, polio, pneumonia.

## 6.3 Ecotoxicology and biomagnification

**Ecotoxicology** is the study of the effects of toxic chemicals, especially at the population, ecosystem, and biosphere levels.

- **Pollutants**: Elements, molecules and particles involved in pollutants which harms life when comes in contact. Pollutants can be introduced naturally or by humans.
- **Poison**: Any substance harmful to body when inhaled, swallowed, injected or in touch to skin. Poisons can be prescribed or OTC medicines having too high doses.
- **Toxins**: Substances which are released into environment by human activities. Carcinogens, mutagens, allergens, neurotransmitters and endocrine disruptors are all toxins.
- **Point sources**: The location is exactly known. Regulated by federal and state agencies. The main point sources are factories and sewage treatments.
- **Non-point sources**: These are the sources of pollution from larger areas rather than a specific point. Runoff is generally associated with non-point source pollution as water is emptied into streams and rivers after accumulating contaminants.
- **Organic**: Polychlorinated biphenyls are present in environment. Aquatic species have higher PCB specifically shown in fish farming.
- **Inorganic**: Heavy metals, pesticides, herbicides, insecticides.
- **Organismic level toxicity:**
- Dermal toxicity on exposure to gasoline.
- Blood toxicity: hypoxia on exposure to CO, leukaemia on exposure to benzene.

- Eye toxicity: acids cause severe nerve corrosion, methanol damages optic nerve.
- Hepatotoxicity: chemical hepatitis, hepatic necrosis, hepatic cancer, cirrhosis, hypersensitivity.
- Neurotoxicity: neuropathies, axonopathies, demyelination, interferon with neurotransmission.
- Nephrotoxicity: inability to excrete body waste, inability to maintain fluid and electrolyte balance, decrease in certain hormones.
- Reproductive toxicity: decreased libido, impotence, interrupted pregnancies, altered sex ratio, multiple births, chromosome abnormalities, birth defects.
- Respiratory toxicity: pulmonary irritation, asthma, bronchitis, emphysema, allergic alveolitis, pneumoconiosis, lung cancer, fibrotic lung disease.

Table 6.1 Natural chemical toxins:

| **Chemical groups** | **Common sources** | **Mode of action** |
|---|---|---|
| Polycyclic Aromatic Hydrocarbons | Bush fires, fuel emission | Carcinogen |
| Biological toxins | Bacteria, fungus, blue green algae | Gastrointestinal, narcotics, neurotoxic |
| Inorganic (CO, CO2, NO2, SH2, NH3) | Volcanic eruption, coal and vehicle emissions | Biochemical pathway blocking |
| Metallic (As, Cd, Cr, Cu, Hg, Pb, Sn, Sb, Zn) | Mining, smelters, paints, batteries, herbicides | Neurotoxic, respiratory blockage. |
| Phenolic compounds | Plant wastes, disinfectants | Cell inhibitors |

Table 6.2 Artificial chemical toxins:

| Chemical groups | Common sources | Mode of action |
|---|---|---|
| Anilines | Dyes | Oxidation, dehydrogenation |
| Antibiotics | Herbicides, biocides | Amino acids inhibitor |
| Benzoylureas | Insecticides | Chitin synthesis inhibitors |
| DDT | Insecticides | Neurotoxic |
| Narcotics | Pharmaceutical industries | Neurotoxic |
| Organochlorides | Fungicides | Neurotoxic: GABA receptors |
| Organometallics | Biocides | Neurotoxic: acetylcholine esterase inhibitors |
| Organophosphorus | Insecticides, herbicides | Unknown |

**Biomagnification:**

- Also known as bio-amplification. Any concentration of toxins present in tissues of organisms which increases successively in higher levels of food chain.
- This increase can occur as a result of:
    - Persistence – where the substance cannot be broken down by environmental processes.
    - Food chain energetics – where the substance's concentration increases progressively as it moves up a food chain.
    - Low or non-existent rate of internal degradation or excretion of the substance – mainly due to water-insolubility.

**Causes of biomagnification:**

- Chemical used in the agriculture sector are highly toxic. Herbicides, insecticides, fungicides. Become a part of the run-off and moves to rivers, oceans.
- Toxic by-products from industries, gas emissions from industrial factories.
- Organic substance like manures, biosolids contains carbon, nitrogen, phosphorus. But these used by industries causes biomagnification.
- Mining by-products like copper, cobalt, zinc, lead get deposited in rivers and waters and leads to biomagnification.

**Novel organic substances** which biomagnify are: DDT, HCB, PCB, toxaphene, monomethyl mercury.

- Mercury is found in small quantity in ocean. Human interference causes an increase of mercury in oceans.
- Algae consistently absorbs the mercury found in its environment. Zoo planktons absorb the algae along with the mercury.
- Small fishes consume large fishes. These are fishes having mercury are consumed by humans which causes illness.
- Biomagnification causes retardation in infants as they contract it from their mothers.
- Also weak immune system occurs.
- Organ failures occur in both animals and humans.

**Prevention of biomagnification:**

- In an attempt to decrease biomagnification, several countries have put a ban on use of DDT.
- Oil and water wastes should be avoided from dropping in water reservoirs.
- Landfills should also be get rid of because these substances seep into the ground water.

### 6.4 Toxicovigilance

- Active process of identifying and evaluating toxic risks in a community and evaluating the measures taken to reduce or to eliminate it.
- The National Poisons Information Centre (NPIC) was established in the department of Pharmacology in AIIMS in 1995.
- Capturing the poisonous cases from intensive and acute medical care units, general acid and emergency departments, casualty at all public healthcare centres.
- Getting poisonous cases from local and overseas media report plays main role for a better understanding of poisoning cases.
- Use of computerized lab data as a detection support tool of toxic reactions in hospitals plays major role in risk factor identification.
- It can also reveal whether there is an emerging toxicological problem resulting from for example: the reformulation of a product or a change from its packaging or labelling, the availability of a new drug of abuse or an environmental contamination.
- Once the poison is identified, the centre is responsible for alerting appropriate health and other authorities.
- Toxicovigilance in laboratory: Identify the poisonous case, collect the data, analyse the data, process-evaluate-communicate and alert authorities as well as public for the prevention actions.

**Multiple Choice Questions:**

**1.** कासप्रतिश्यायशिरोरुजश्च भवन्तितीव्रा नयनामायाश्च।। **.... is the Vishakta Lakshana of?**

A. Vayu B. Jala C. Bhumi D. Kala

**2. Acid rain depletes which nutrition?**
A. Zinc B. Magnesium C. Aluminium D. Calcium

**3. The Minimata incident of Japan happened in which year?**
A. 1950 B. 1982 C. 1932 D. 1921

**4. Which plant absorbs dissolved toxic chemicals like cadmium?**
A. Oak B. Water hyacinth C. Banyan D. Neem

**5. Anthrax is caused by....?**
A. Variola major B. Yersinia pestis
C. Burkholderia D. Bacillus anthracis

**6. First deal between Germans & French not to use poisonous bullets was done in which yea?**
A. 1675 B. 1155 C. 1650 D. 1863

**7. Entomological warfare is a biological war using what?**
A. Poison B. Insects C. Bullets D. Virus

**8. Which of the following is a choking chemical agent?**
A. Nitrogen mustard B. Hydrogen cyanide
C. Lewisite D. Chloropicrin

**9. Atomic bombs were dropped in Hiroshima in which year?**
A. 1945 B. 1917 C. 1965 D. 1999

**10. Which of the following is an artificial chemical toxin?**
A. CO B. Cr C. DDT D. Zn

**11. Novel organic substance which biomagnifies is?**
A. Organochlorides B. Antibiotics C. Toxaphene D. Anilines

**12. Concentration of toxins present in tissues of organisms which increases successively in higher levels of food chain. ... is known as?**

A. Ecotoxicology
B. Chemical warfare
C. Biological warfare
D. Biomagnification

**13. Which is the long term effect of nuclear warfare?**

A. Erythema
B. Sterility
C. Peri-natal mortality
D. Low sperm count

**14. The study of the effects of toxic chemicals, especially at the population, ecosystem, and biosphere levels.... Is called as?**

A. Ecotoxicology
B. Chemical warfare
C. Biological warfare
D. Biomagnification

**15. Which of the following is a natural chemical toxin?**

A. Benzoylureas
B. DDT
C. Polycyclic aromatic hydrocarbons
D. Anilines

**Answer key for MCQs:**

| | |
|---|---|
| 1 | A |
| 2 | D |
| 3 | C |
| 4 | B |
| 5 | D |
| 6 | A |
| 7 | B |
| 8 | D |

| | |
|---|---|
| 9 | A |
| 10 | C |
| 11 | C |
| 12 | D |
| 13 | C |
| 14 | A |
| 15 | C |

# Ch. 7
# Dermatological Manifestation of Visha

### 7.1 Contact dermatitis and its Management

The dermatological manifestation can vary widely depending on the poison involved, route of ingestion, duration of exposure, various individual factors. Poisoning can be by ingesting, inhaling, injecting or skin contact. The most common manifestation of poisoning occurs:

- **Rash**: The poisoning can cause various developments on skin like hives, red bumps, red patches. The appearance of rash depends on toxic substances.
- **Skin irritation**: Redness, itching, irritation can be caused by poison contact. It can occur due to irritant chemicals like acids or industrial chemicals.
- **Blisters**: Certain chemicals or toxins can cause the formation of blisters on skin. It can be filled with clear fluid, blood or pus.
- **Burns**: Strong acids, base or corrosives causes chemical burns on skin. These require special medical treatments.
- **Hypo pigmentation**: Some chemicals or toxics exposure cause loss in normal skin pigmentation and causes white patches.
- **Hyper pigmentation**: Some chemicals or toxins on exposure causes darkening or discoloration of the affected area.
- **Pruritus**: Itching is the most common manifestation in poisoning contact and it can be much distressing.
- **Ulcerations**: Severe poisoning can cause skin ulcers or open sores. These are painful and slow in healing.

- Pesticides can also injure the skin directly known as cutaneous toxicity.
- The degree of inflammation is a direct result of degree of physical or chemical irritation.
- If there is severe damage, resulting in cell death than skin can become denuded which is loss of layers of skin causing deeper layers to get exposed.
- Allergic dermatitis caused by poisonous oak is the most frequent cause of temporary disability in forestry workers.

Table 7.1 Pesticides causing dermatitis

| | | |
|---|---|---|
| Sulphur | Omite | Weed oil |
| Captafol | Folpate | Dacthal |
| Endosulphan | Lindane | Chlorothalonil |
| Toxaphene | Ziram | Organophosphates |
| Chloropicrin | Thiram | Maneb |

Table 7.2 Plants causing dermatitis:

| | | |
|---|---|---|
| Tomatoes | Carrot | Castor bean |
| Mushrooms | Daffodil | Cucumber |
| Parsnip | Turnip | Tulip bulb |
| Parsley | Celery | Butter cup |
| Rubber tree | Foxglove | Milk weed |

7.3 Pesticides causing Allergic Contact Dermatitis:

| | |
|---|---|
| TOK | Malathion |
| Cresol | Triazine |
| PCNB | Benomyl |
| Naled | Natural pyrethroids |

7.4 Flower plants causing Allergic Contact Dermatitis:

| Poison Ivy | Chrysanthemum |
|---|---|
| Poison oak | Primrose |
| English Ivy | Tulip bulbs |
| Cedar | Lichens |
| Pine | Cashew sumac |

***Treatment:***

- Removal of the irritant by washing avoid further contact with the chemical.
- 0.5% hydrocortisone may help alleviate pain and itching.
- Prevent the exposure to chemical containing areas.
- Protective equipment be used by the forestry workers to avoid contact.
- Immunosuppressant, anti histamine medications be used.
- Washing hands after immediately coming in contact with the chemicals.
- Large blisters when break, care be taken to avoid secondary infections.
- Benzocaine containing creams be avoided as they can act as contact sanitizers.

**7.2 Signs, Symptoms and Management of Abhyanga visha, Lepa visha, Vastra visha, Paduka visha, Abharana visha with Contemporary Relevance**

- मुखगत विष ( poison in mouth):

    स चेत् प्रमादान्मोहाद्वा तदन्नमुपसेवते।

    अष्ठीलावत्ततो जिह्वा भवत्यरसवेदिनी ।। (सु.क. १/३८)

If poisoned food intaken the tongue becomes hard, incapable to recognize taste, burning sensation, more saliva flows out.

**Treatment:** Treatment suggested in poisoned fumes and incision done on swelling and applied with Dhataki pushpa, Pathya, Jambu seeds with Kshaudra. Paste of roots of Ankota mixed with honey, bark of Saptachhada with honey, seeds of Shirisha with honey.

- आमाशयगत विष (poison in small intestine):

मूर्च्छा छर्दिमतीसारमाध्मानं दाहवेपथू ।
इन्द्रियाणां च वैकृत्यं कुर्यादामाशयं गतम् ।।
तत्राशु मदनालाबुबिम्बीकोशातकीफलैः ।
छर्दनं दध्युदश्विद्भ्यामथवा तण्डुलाम्बुना ।। (सु.क. १/४०–४१)

Poison entering small intestine causes vomiting, diarrhoea, flatulence, fainting, shivering, disorder of sense organs.

**Treatment:** Vamana should be done by administering powder of Madana, Bimbi, Alabu, Koshthaki mixed with curd, diluted buttermilk or rice wash.

- पक्वाशयगत विष (poison in large intestine):

दाहं मूर्च्छामतीसारं तृष्णामिन्द्रियवैकृतम् ।
आटोपं पाण्डुतां कार्श्यं कुर्यात् पक्वाशयं गतम् ।।
विरेचनं ससर्पिष्कं तत्रोक्तं नीलिनीफलम् ।
दध्ना दूषीविषारिश्च पेयो वा मधुसंयुतः ।। (सु.क. १/४२–४३)

Poison reaching large intestine causes burning sensation, fainting, diarrhoea, thirst, disorder of the senses, gurgling of abdomen, yellowish discoloration, emaciation.

**Treatment:** Virechana be done using Niliniphala with Ghee or Dooshivishari Agada with curd.

- दन्तकाष्ठ विष (poison in toothbrush):

विशीर्यते कूर्चकस्तु दन्तकाष्ठगते विषे ।
जिह्वादन्तौष्ठमांसानां श्वयथुश्चोपजायते ।।
अथास्य धातकीपुष्पपथ्याजम्बूफलास्थिभिः ।
सक्षौद्रैः प्रच्छिते शोफे कर्तव्यं प्रतिसारणम् ।।
अथवाऽङ्कोठमूलानि त्वचः सप्तच्छदस्य वा ।

शिरीषमाषका वाऽपि सक्षौद्राः प्रतिसारणम्।। (सु.क.१/४८–५०)

Poisoned toothbrush looses its bristles, swelling of tongue, teeth, gums, lips.

**Treatment:** Incision done on swelling and applied with Dhataki pushpa, Pathya, Jambu seeds with Kshaudra. Paste of roots of Ankota mixed with honey, bark of Saptachhada with honey, seeds of Shirisha with honey.

- जिह्वानिर्लेखक विष (poison in tongue cleanser):

जिह्वानिर्लेखकवलौ दन्तकाष्ठवदादिशेत् । (सु.क.१/५१)

Poisoned toothbrush looses its bristles, swelling of tongue, teeth, gums, lips.

**Treatment:** Incision done on swelling and applied with Dhataki pushpa, Pathya, Jambu seeds with Kshaudra. Paste of roots of Ankota mixed with honey, bark of Saptachhada with honey, seeds of Shirisha with honey.

- अभ्यंगविष (poisonous massage):

पिच्छिलो बहुलोऽभ्यङ्गो विवर्णो वा विषान्वितः।।<br>
स्फोटजन्मरुजास्रावत्वक्पाकः स्वेदनं ज्वरः।<br>
दरणं चापि मांसानामभ्यङ्गे विषसंयुते।।<br>
तत्र शीताम्बुसिक्तस्य कर्तव्यमनुलेपनम्।<br>
चन्दनं तगरं कुष्ठमुशीरं वेणुपत्रिका।।<br>
सोमवल्ल्यमृता श्वेता पद्मं कालीयकं त्वचम्।<br>
कपित्थरसमूत्राभ्यां पानमेतच्च युज्यते।। (सु.क.१/५१–५४)

Poisonous oil for massage is slimy, when used produces eruptions, spots, pain, exudations, ulcers, excess sweating, fever.

**Treatment:** Pour cold water on body. Apply paste of Chandana, Tagara, Kushtha, Ushira, Venupatra, Somavalli, Amruta, Shveta, Padma, Kaliyaka. Drinking water should also be processed with these drugs.

- मुखलेपगत विष (poison in Lepa):

    मुखालेपे मुखं श्यावं युक्तमभ्यङ्गलक्षणैः।
    पद्मिनीकण्टकप्रख्यैः कण्टकैश्चोपचीयते।।
    तत्र क्षौद्रघृतं पानं प्रलेपश्चन्दनं घृतम्।
    पयस्या मधुकं फञ्जी बन्धुजीवः पुनर्नवा।। (सु.क.१/६०–६१)

Gives blackish discoloration to face. Face gets covered with eruptions like those in lotus called as Padmini kantaka.

**Treatment:** Drink ghee and honey. Apply paste of Chandana, Payasya, Madhuka, Phanji, Bandhujihva, Punarnava mixed with ghee.

- नस्यधूमगत विष (poison in Nasya and Dhooma):

    शोणितागमनं खेभ्यः शिरोरुक्कफसंस्रवः।।
    नस्यधूमगते लिङ्गमिन्द्रियाणां च वैकृतम्।
    तत्र दुग्धैर्गवादीनां सर्पिः सातिविषैः श्रृतम्।। (सु.क.१/६३–६४)

Bleeding from orifices, headache, more flow of Kapha, disorder of the sense organs.

**Treatment:** Milk or ghee boiled with Ativisha, Shveta, Madyantika should be used in drinking and as nasal drops.

- पादुकाविष (poison in footwear):

    शोफः स्रावस्तथा स्वापः पादयोः स्फोटजन्म च।।
    भवन्ति विषजुष्टाभ्यां पादुकाभ्यामसंशयम्।
    उपानत्पादपीठानि पादुकावत् प्रसाधयेत्।। (सु.क.१/७२–७३)

Footwear poison causes swelling, exudation, loss of sensation, eruptions. These similar symptoms occur in poisoned foot rest and pillows.

- आभारण विष (poison in ornament)

भूषणानि हतार्चींषि न विभान्ति यथा पुरा।
स्वानि स्थानानि हन्युश्च दाहपाकावदारणैः।। (सु.क.१/७४)

The ornaments lose their shine and brightness. The places they touch cause burning, ulcerations, bruising.

## 7.3 Signs, Symptoms and Management of Dermatological Manifestations due to Cosmetics, Chemicals, Occupational and other Allergens

**1. Irritant dermatitis:** Facial cleansers: these often contain surfactants that are necessary to clean the skin.

- Toners and astringents: these may contain alcohol or acids such as alpha-hydroxyacid (AHA), which can cause skin problems in some people.
- Facial treatment: this involves the use of manual manipulation and application of chemicals on the skin, often resulting in exfoliation of the upper skin surface. Mild irritation is inevitable, but severe skin inflammation like dermatitis can occur.

**Signs and symptoms:**

- Burning, tingling sensation, itchiness, redness, swelling. Later scaling and peeling of skin can occur.

**Treatment:**

- Stop using all cosmetic products on the affected skin immediately.
- After the rash has cleared, patch testing may be required at a later date to exclude an allergy to the cosmetics.

**2. Dermatitis due to chemicals:**

- Manufacturing chemicals is important for various industries like agriculture but takes a toll on workers.
- Uneven safety regulations through out the global chemical

industry increases the risk.

- **Contact dermatitis:** The hands are affected the most. Other sites are wrists, forearms, face, neck. Acute presentation may be swelling, blisters. Chronic may show fissured dry or scaly lesions.
- **Follicular lesions:** Oil folliculitis occurs due to cutting oil and tar products. Chlorine based chemicals causes chloracne.
- **Skin cancer:** Skin lesions due to exposure to polycyclic hydrocarbons. Lesions may not appear until decades after the exposure.
- **Chemical burns:** Solvents, acids, alkalis, detergents, oxidising agents cause the harm.
- **Contact leukoderma:** White patches are shown if skin comes in contact with phenolic compounds.

**Diagnosis:**

- Based on clinical symptoms and signs.
- Appearance, location and course of lesions.
- Occupational history of the patient. Duration, exposure and time length of exposure during working hours.
- Patch test if contact allergy is suspected.
- Biopsy if needed.

**Treatment:**

- Topical corticosteroids
- Oral prednisolone
- Gloves, goggles, eye protectors, respiratory masks, chemo protective clothing.
- Applying moisturizers as needed.
- Use of personal protective equipment.

**3. Occupational dermatitis:**

***A. Contact phototoxic photo sensitization:***

- Most common occupational photo toxic reaction in humans

caused primarily by plants.

- Occurs when photo active chemicals or fungus contacts the skin, absorbed into the skin and then activated by sunlight.

**Symptoms:** Redness, pain, blistering, hyper pigmentation of the affected area following recovery.

Table 7.5 Plants causing photo sensitization

| | |
|---|---|
| Figs | Buttercup |
| Dill | Parsley |
| Mustard | Carrots |
| Lime | Celery with pink rot |

***B. Photo allergic photoreaction:***

- Very similar to contact dermatitis.
- Here, sunlight is very important to initiate the process.
- Requires prior exposure to chemicals followed by sunlight. Though this is not very common.
- Clothing and application of sunscreen helps to prevent the condition.

## 7.4 Dermatological manifestation due to Dooshivisha and Garavisha

***A. Dermatological manifestation due to Dooshivisha:***

- The artificial poison vitiates blood and produces eczema, psoriasis, boils on head, urticaria.
- Acne & pimples: The accumulation of toxins in body can lead to Dosha vitiation and leads to acne & pimples.
- Eczema: Dooshivisha disrupts skin's natural balance and leads to inflammation causing eczema.
- Psoriasis: Accumulation of toxins can trigger the immune response that affects skin and potentially causes psoriasis.
- Hives: Accumulated toxins causes allergic reactions which disrupts the normal immune system and leads to hives.

- Dermatitis: Imbalanced Doshas and accumulation of toxins leads to various forms of dermatitis, skin inflammation, irritation.
- Rashes: Skin rashes including contact dermatitis can be associated with imbalance and toxins in the body.
- Pruritus: Itchy skin can be a common symptom of Dooshivisha related dermatological problems.

**Treatment:**

- Commonly involves the purification of body by Panchakarma therapies like Vamana, Virechana.
- Lifestyle and dietary modification, herbal remedies are used to restore the natural balance of Doshas and to eliminate toxins from the body.

***B. Dermatological manifestation due to Garavisha:***

- Allergic reactions: Exposure to toxins or allergens in environment can lead to allergic reactions.
- Contact dermatitis: Contact with toxic substances can cause redness, itching, blisters on skin.
- Eczema: Garavisha can trigger the eczema leading to skin inflammation, dryness, itching.
- Skin rashes: Resulting from the toxic plant exposure can occur due to Garavisha.
- Photosensitivity: Some toxins can make skin more sensitive to sunlight leading to sunburn.
- Vitiligo: Garavisha sometimes leads to toxic manifestations like vitiligo.
- Acne & boils: Impurities in body can disrupt the normal balance of Doshas leading to skin conditions like acne & boils.

**Treatment:**

- Commonly involves the purification of body by Panchakarma therapies like Vamana, Virechana.

- Lifestyle and dietary modification, herbal remedies are used to restore the natural balance of Doshas and to eliminate toxins from the body.

## 7.5 Dermatological Manifestation due to Bites and Stings

- Sarpa Visha (Snake poison): Inflammation, blackish discoloration at site of bite, raised site of bite, pain, burning sensation.
- Kita Visha (Insect venom): Inflammation, itching, discharge, skin eruptions.
- Makshika Visha (Bee venom): Itching, Burning sensation, swelling, pain, skin eruptions.
- Kanabha Visha: Blackish discoloration at the site of bite, inflammation, severe pain.
- Manduka Visha (Frog venom): Burning, itching.
- Gruhagodhika Visha (Lizard venom): Pain like a needle prick, burning sensation.
- Pipilika Visha (Ant venom): Burning sensation, swelling like the touch of fire.
- Mashaka Visha (Mosquito bite): Intense itching, swelling at the site of bite.
- Luta Visha (Spider venom): Rashes, swelling, pain, bleeding, herpes at 10 places.
- Vrushchika Visha (Scorpion venom): Burning sensation, piercing pricking pain, blackening at the site of bite.
- Mushaka Visha (Rat poison): Moistness, inflammation.
- Alarka Visha: Numbness at the site of bite, itching, pain, eruptions, formation of blisters and later on rupture.

**Multiple Choice Questions:**

**1. Which plant doesn't cause photo sensitization?**

A. Buttercup B. Fig C. Lime D. Neem

**2. Thiram comes under which category of causing dermatitis?**
A. Pesticides B. Flowers C. Plants D. Fruits

**3. Which of the following plant does not cause dermatitis?**
A. Tomatoes B. Radish C. Carrots D. Celery

**4. Niliniphala Ghrita should be given to treat poisoning of which organ?**
A. Small intestine B. Mouth C. Large intestine D. Tongue

**5. In which type of poisoning does the face get covered with eruptions like Padmini Kantaka?**
A. Abhyanga B. Nasya C. Dhooma D. Lepa

**6. Contact leukoderma due to contact with which compound?**
A. Chlorine B. Phenolic compounds
C. Sulphuric acid D. Alkalis

**7. Herpes at 10 sites of body is a dermatologic manifestation due to which poisonous sting?**
A. Luta B. Mooshika C. Kanabha D. Mashaka

**8. Chloracne occurs due to which substance?**
A. Phenolic compounds B. Alkalis
C. Chlorine D. Sulphuric acid

**9. Burning sensation like the touch of fire is the dermatologic manifestation of which sting?**
A. Makshika B. Kanabha C. Gruhagodhika D. Pipilika

**10.** पिच्छिलो बहुलोऽभ्यङ्गो विवर्णो वा विषान्वितः || **...... is the Shloka for poisoning in?**
A. Paduka B. Abhyanga C. Dhooma D. Nasya

**Answer key for MCQs:**

| | |
|---|---|
| 1 | D |
| 2 | A |
| 3 | B |
| 4 | C |
| 5 | D |

| | |
|---|---|
| 6 | B |
| 7 | A |
| 8 | C |
| 9 | D |
| 10 | B |

# Ch. 8
# Therapeutic Utility of Agada Yoga

## 8.1 Dooshivishari Agada

दूषीविषार्तं सुस्विन्नमूर्ध्वं चाधश्च शोधितम्।
पाययेतागदं नित्यमिमं दूषीविषापहम्।।
पिप्पल्यो ध्यामकं मांसी शावरः परिपेलवम्।
सुवर्चिका ससूक्ष्मैला तोयं कनकगैरिकम्।।
क्षौद्रयुक्तोऽगदो ह्येष दूषीविषमपोहति।
नाम्ना दूषीविषारिस्तु न चान्यत्रापि वार्यते।। (सु.क.५०–५२)

The person suffering from Dooshivisha should be given Swedana. Later Vamana and Virechana should be given. Followed by giving Agad to remove the poisonous effects.

| Ingredients | |
|---|---|
| Pippali | Piper longum |
| Dhyamaka | Cymbopogon martinii |
| Jatamamsi | Nardostachys jatamamsi |
| Lodhra | Symplococus racemosa |
| Ela | Elettaria cardomomum |
| Suvarchika | Salt petre |
| Kutannatum | Oroxylim indicum |
| Natam | Valeriana wallichii |
| Kushtha | Saussurea lappa |
| Yashtimadhu | Glycyrrhiza glabra |
| Chandana | Santalum album |
| Gairik | Red ochre |

**Anupana:** Madhu.
**Indications:** Dooshivisha.

### 8.2 Bilwadi Agada

बिल्वस्य मूलं सुरसस्य पुष्पं फलं करञ्जस्य नतं सुराह्वम्।
फलत्रिकं व्योषनिशाद्वयं च वस्तस्य मूत्रेण सुसूक्ष्मपिष्टम।।
भुजङ्गलूतोन्दुरवृश्चिकाद्यैर्विसूचिकाजीर्णगरज्वरैश्च।
आर्तान्नरान् भूतविधर्षितांश्च स्वस्थीकरोत्यञ्जनपाननस्यैः।।
(अ.हृ.उ. ३६/८४–८५)

**Ingredients:** Roots of Bilwa, flowers of Surasa, fruits of Karanja, Nata, Surahvam, Phalatrika, Vyosha, two types of Nisha.

All the above ingredients should be macerated in goat's urine and made into a fine paste.

**Indications:** Used as Anjana (Collyrium), Pana (internally), Nasya (nasal drops). It is useful in the cure of poisonous bites of Sarpa (snake), Luta (spiders), Mooshaka (rats), Vrushchika (scorpion). Also useful in Vishuchika (vomiting and diarrhoea), Ajirna (indigestion), Jwara (fever).

### 8.3 Dashanga Agada

वचा हिङ्गु विडङ्गानि सैन्धवं गजपिप्पली।।
पाठा प्रतिविषा व्योषं काश्यपेन विनिर्मितम्।
दशाङ्गमगदं पीत्वा सर्वकीटविषं जयेत।।
(अ.हृ.उ. ३७/२७–२८)

**Ingredients:** Vacha, Hingu, Vidanga, Saindhava, Gajapippali, Patha, Prativisha, Vyosha. These should be made into small pills.

**Indications:** The Agada formed by Acharya Kashyapa cures the poisons of all kinds of insect bites.

### 8.4 Murvadi Agada:

मूर्वामृतानतकणापटोलीचव्यचित्रकान् ।।
वचामुस्तविडङ्गानि तक्रकोष्णाम्बुमस्तुभिः ।
पिबेद्रसेन वाऽम्लेन गरोपहतपावकः ।। (अ.हृ.उ. ३७ / ५७–५८)

Ingredients: Powder of Murva, Amruta, Nata, Kana, Patoli, Chitraka, Vacha, Musta, Vidanga. These should be mixed with either Takra, Ushna jala, Mastu, meat soup or sour liquid.

Indications: It is very useful in person who has Agni mandya due to Garavisha.

### 8.5 Panchashirisha Agada:

शिरीषफलमूलत्वक्पुष्पपत्रैः समैर्धृतैः ।
श्रेष्ठः पञ्चशिरीषोऽयं विषाणां प्रवरो वध ।।
इति पञ्चशिरीषोऽगदः । (च.चि.२३ / २१८)

The Panchanga of Shirisha as Phala, Moola, Twaka, Pushpa, Patra be taken in equal quantity is called as Pancha Shirisha Agada.

Ingredients: This is one among the best formulations for treating poison.

### 8.6 Vishaghna Mahakashaya (Charak Samhita):

हरिद्रामञ्जिष्ठासुवहासूक्ष्मैलापालिन्दीचन्दनकतकशिरीषसिन्धुवारश्लेष्मातका इति दशेमानि विषघ्नानि भवन्ति ।।
(च.सू. ४ / ११ / १६)

| Ingredients | |
|---|---|
| Haridra | Curcuma longa |
| Manjishtha | Rubia cordifolia |
| Suvaha | Operculina turpethum |
| Sukshma Ela | Elettaria cardomomum |

| Palindi | Ichnocarpus frutescens |
|---|---|
| Chandana | Santalum album |
| Kataka | Strychnos potatorium |
| Shirisha | Albizzia lebbeck |
| Sindhuvara | Vitex negundo |
| Shleshmatak | Cordia dichotama |

**Indications:** These 10 drugs cure Visha Roga. This is one among the best formulations for treating poison.

### 8.7 Ekasara Gana (Sushruta Samhita):

सोमराजीफलं पुष्पं कटभी सिन्धुवारकः।
चोरको वरुणः कुष्ठं सर्पगन्धा ससप्तला।।
पुनर्नवा शिरीषस्य पुष्पमारग्वधार्कजम।
श्यामाऽम्बष्ठा विडङ्गानि तथाऽम्राश्मन्तकानि च।
भूमी कुरबकश्चैव गण एकसरः स्मृतः।
एकशो द्वित्रिशो वाऽपि प्रयोक्तव्यो विषापहः।।
(सु.क. ५/ ८४–८६)

Fruits and flowers of Somaraji, Katabhi, Sindhuvarak, Choraka, Varuna, Kushtha, Sarpagnadha, Saptala, Punarnava, flowers of Shirisha-Aragwadha-Arka, Shyama, Ambashtha, Vidanga, Amra, Ashmantaka, Bhumi and Kurabaka. Together these are called as Ekasara Gana.

**Indications:** These ingredients can be used individually or in combination of 2-3 drugs to destroy the poison. This is one among the best formulations for treating poison.

**Multiple Choice Questions**

**1. What is the Latin name of Suvaha?**

A. Santalum album B. Operculina turpethum
C. Vitex negundo D. Curcuma longa

**2. Bilwadi Agada is not mentioned for which procedure?**

A. Pana B. Nasya C. Abhyanga D. Anjana

**3. Panchashirisha Agada is mentioned in which chapter by Acharya Charak?**

A. 23 B. 25 C. 21 D. 27

**4. What is the Latin name for Kushtha?**

A. Oroxylim indicum B. Piper longum
C. Symplococus racemosa D. Saussurea lappa

**5. What is the Anupana for Dooshivishari Agada?**

A. Jala B. Madhu C. Takra D. Sura

**Answer key for MCQs:**

| 1 | B |
|---|---|
| 2 | C |
| 3 | A |
| 4 | D |
| 5 | B |

# Ch. 9
# Sthavara Visha: Poisons of Plant Origin

## 1. Cardiac Poisons

- *Vatsanabha:*
    - **Botanical name:** Aconitum ferox, Aconitum napellus.
    - **Family:** Ranunculaceae
    - **Varga:** Visha Varga
    - **Kula:** Vatsanabha Kula
    - **Type of poison:** Cardiac poison
    - **Synonyms:** Aconite, Vatsanaga, Monk's hood, Amrura, Kshveda, Garala.
    - **Toxic parts:** Roots being more toxic, seeds.
    - **Toxic principles:** Aconitine, meso-aconitine, hypo-aconitine.
    - **Mechanism of action:** Stimulates vagal medullary centre
    - **Fatal dose:** 1-2gm of roots, 250mg extract, 25 drops of tincture, 4mg alkaloid.
    - **Fatal period:** 20 minutes to 24 hours

Table 9.1

| | |
|---|---|
| **Signs and symptoms** | • Nausea, vomiting, diarrhoea, salivation, tingling and numbness in mouth and lips<br>• Palpitations, weakness, hypotension, arrhythmia, vertigo, convulsions<br>• Blurring of vision, mydriasis, xanthopsia |
| **Management** | • Gastric lavage with activated charcoal<br>• Benzodiazepines for convulsions<br>• Symptomatic treatment<br>• Patola Swarasa with 1 pala sugar |

| Pot mortem appearance | • No specific findings<br>• Organs are congested |
|---|---|
| **Medico-legal aspects** | • Ideal homicidal poisoning as sweet in taste can be given with food.<br>• Suicide<br>• Accidental poisoning<br>• Arrow poison, cattle poison, used to procure abortion. |
| **Therapeutic dose** | • 60 to 125 mg |

Image 9.1 Plant of Vatsanabha

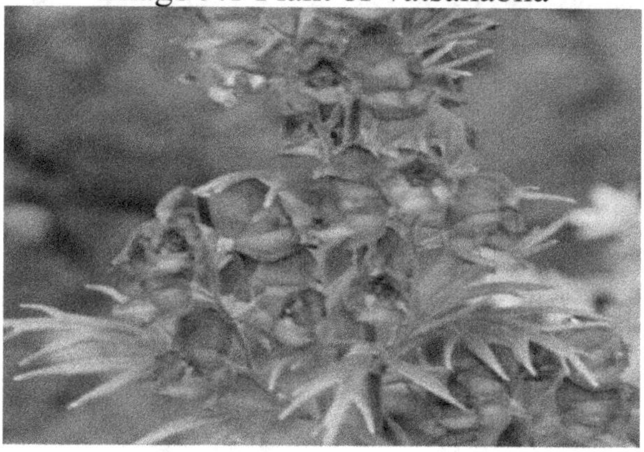

Image 9.2 Bark of Vatsanabha

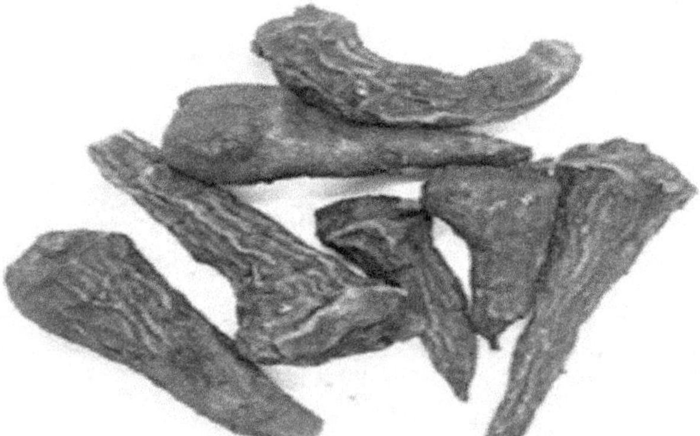

- **Karveera**
  - **Botanical name:** Nerium indicum
  - **Family**: Apocynaceace
  - **Kula**: Kutaja Kula
  - **Types**: Shweta, pita
  - **Synonyms**: Ashwamaraka, Hayamara, Hayamaraka, Chandataka.
  - **Toxic parts**: All parts but root being the most toxic.
  - **Toxic principles**: Oleandrin, neriin, nerifolin, cerberia, folinerin.
  - **Mechanism of action**: Cardiac effects of glycosides are due to direct cardio-toxicity and indirect effect via the vagal nerve.
  - **Fatal dose**: Seeds: 8-10, Twaka churna: 15-20gm, 5-10 leaves.
  - **Fatal period**: 24 hours.

Table 9.2

| | |
|---|---|
| **Signs and symptoms** | • Vomiting, abdominal pain, frothy saliva, restlessness.<br>• Slow and weak pulse, lock jaw.<br>• Exhaustion, drowsiness, coma and lastly death. |
| **Management** | • Gastric lavage by tannic acid. Maintain electrolyte balance and vitals.<br>• Life support system and symptomatic treatment.<br>• Mahisha Dadhi with sugar, Mahisha Dugdha with sugar.<br>• Arka Twaka Churna with water |
| **Post-mortem appearance** | • Haemolysis of RBC, organs congested.<br>• Renal tubes blocked by haemoglobin. |
| **Medico-legal aspects** | • Seeds are used for suicidal poisoning<br>• Roots are used to procure abortion<br>• Cattle poisoning |
| **Therapeutic dose** | • 30 to 125 mg/day |

Image 9.3 Flowers of Karveera

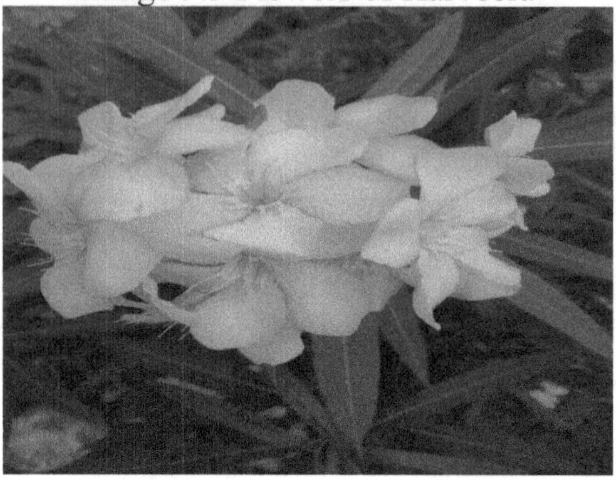

- **Hrutpatti**
  - **Botanical name:** Digitalis purpurea
  - **Family**: Scrophulariaceae
  - **Kula**: Katuka Kula
  - **Types**: Cardiac poison
  - **Synonyms**: Tila pushpi, fox glove, lady's glove, common fox glove, purple fox glove.
  - **Toxic parts**: Leaves
  - **Toxic principles**: Digitalis, digitoxin.
  - **Mechanism of action**: Not much specific. But as suicidal or homicidal and as folk medicine.
  - **Fatal dose**: Digitalis: 2mg, Digitoxin: 3mg
  - **Fatal period**: 30 minutes to 24 hours

Table 9.3

| **Signs and symptoms** | • Vomiting, loss of appetite, contusion, blurred vision.<br>• Changes in colour perception, Xanthopsia, tremors.<br>• Nausea, vomiting, diarrhoea, drooling, weakness, dilated pupil. |
|---|---|

| Management | • Supportive care, activated charcoal.<br>• Atropine<br>• Antidote: Digoxin specific antibody fragments. |
|---|---|
| Post-mortem appearance | • Signs of asphyxia |
| Medico-legal aspects | • Accidental poisoning, stupefying poison. |
| Therapeutic dose | • Leaf powder: 500mg, alcoholic extract: 5-15 mg. |

- **Tobacco**
  - **Botanical name**: Nicotina tabacum
  - **Family**: Solanaceae
  - **Kula**: Kantakari Kula
  - **Types**: Cardiac poison
  - **Synonyms**: Guchhaphala, Galanja, Tamala.
  - **Toxic parts**: Leaves
  - **Toxic principles**: Cerberin, nicotine, nornicotine. Nicotine is colourless, volatile, bitter and hygroscopic liquid.
  - **Mechanism of action**: Nicotine receptors present in CNS, autonomic ganglion, adrenal medulla, spinal cord, chemoreceptors of carotid and aortic bodies.
  - **Fatal dose**: 40-60 mg of Nicotine, 15-30 gm of crude tobacco, 1-2 drops of pure nicotine.
  - **Fatal period**: 5-15 minutes

Table 9.4

| Signs and symptoms | • Nausea, vomiting, severe diarrhoea, abdominal pain, blurred vision, bradycardia, irregular breathing. |
|---|---|
| Acute poisoning | • Nausea, vomiting, diarrhoea, pain in abdomen.<br>• Salivation, blurred vision, anxiety, headache, confusion.<br>• Tachycardia followed by bradycardia.<br>• Convulsions, paralysis, coma. |

| | |
|---|---|
| **Chronic poisoning** | • Found among nicotine addiction, smokers, tobacco chewers.<br>• Recurrent craving for tobacco, cough, impaired memory, amblyopia.<br>• Tobacco withdrawal has mood swings, insomnia, restlessness, constipation, headache, anxiety. |
| **Management** | • Stomach wash, atropine, management of hyperkalaemia. |
| **Post-mortem appearance** | • Signs of asphyxia, brownish froth, congestion of GIT, pulmonary oedema. |
| **Medico-legal aspects** | • Accidental poisoning, malingering, suicidal poisoning, homicidal poisoning, occupational hazard. |
| **Uses** | • Smoking tobacco, chewing, snuff, insecticide. |
| **Therapeutic dose** | • 1 to 2 gm |
| **Complications** | • Carcinoma of lung, oesophagus, pharynx, mouth.<br>• Smoker's cough, bronchitis.<br>• Thromboangitis obliterans, tobacco amblyopia. |
| **Maternal smoking effects** | • Increased risk of spontaneous abortion, placenta previa, abruptio placentae.<br>• Fetal death, low birth weight baby. |

- **Cerebra odollam:**
  - **Botanical name**: Cerebra odollam
  - **Family**: Apocynacaea
  - **Toxic parts**: Fruits
  - **Toxic principles**: Cerberin.
  - **Mechanism of action**: The kernels of C. Odollam contains cerebrin a digoxin type cardenolide and cardiac glycoside that blocks the calcium ion channels in heart muscles causing disruption of heartbeat most often fatally.
  - **Fatal dose**: Kernel of 1 fruit
  - **Fatal period**: 1-2 days

Table 9.5

| | |
|---|---|
| **Signs and symptoms** | • Nausea, vomiting, abdominal pain, diarrhoea.<br>• Irregular breathing, bradycardia, bitter taste in mouth.<br>• Collapse, death. |
| **Management** | • Gastric lavage<br>• IV molar solution of sodium lactate to combat acidosis.<br>• 5% glucose solution with 1.2 mg of atropine.<br>• 2ml of adrenaline 1:1000 and 2mg of nor adrenaline to combat heart block.<br>• Symptomatic treatment. |
| **Post-mortem appearance** | • Signs of GIT irritation and congestion of organs. |
| **Medico-legal aspects** | • Accidental poisoning, homicidal poisoning, poisoning to commit suicide in dowry cases. |
| **Therapeutic dose** | • Used as external application. |

Image 9.4 Kernel of Cerebra odollam

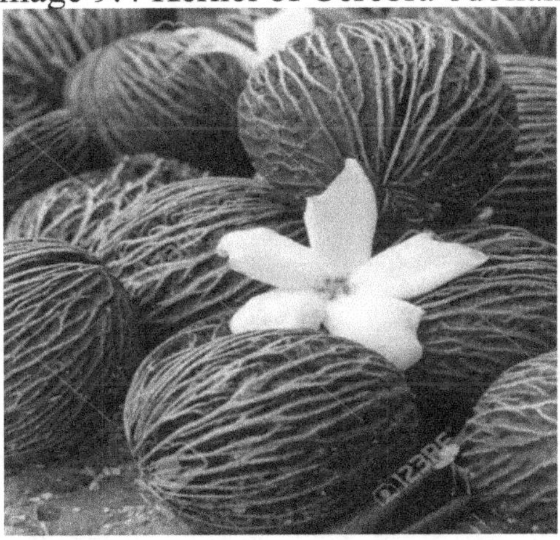

## 2. Neurotoxic poisons:

- Kupeelu:
    - **Botanical name**: Strychnos nux vomica
    - **Family**: Loganiaceae
    - **Kula**: Karashara Kula

- **Varieties**: Strychnos wallichiana, Strychnos ignatti
- **Type**: Neurotoxic poison
- **Synonyms**: Vishamooshika, Vishatinduka, Kakapilu, Dog buttons.
- **Toxic parts**: Seed, bark
- **Toxic principles**: Seed contains Strychnine, Brucine. Root, stem, bark, leaves contain Brucine and Lagonin.
- Absorption is from GI mucosa and nasal mucosa.
- Metabolism occurs in liver.
- Excretion is from kidney and traces from bile, milk, saliva.
- **Mechanism of action**: Strychnine antagonizes the inhibitory neurotransmitter amino acid glycine at post synaptic receptors.
- **Fatal dose**: 1-2 crushed seeds, strychnine 50-100 mg.
- **Fatal period**: 1-2 hours

Table 9.6

| | |
|---|---|
| **Signs and symptoms** | • Stiffness: Spasms of jaw and neck.<br>• Twiching, back stiffness, convulsions, breathlessness. |
| **Complications** | • Hypoxia, hyperthermia, rhabdomyolysis.<br>• Metabolic acidosis, lactic acidosis. |
| **Causes of death** | • Medullary paralysis, respiratory. |
| **Differential diagnosis** | • Rabies, Tetanus, Meningitis, Cocaine intoxication, hysteria. |
| **Management** | • Patient be managed in calm environment.<br>• Benzodiazepines for convulsions.<br>• Activated charcoal, symptomatic treatment. |
| **Post-mortem appearance** | • Rigor mortis<br>• Post mortem caloricity, signs of asphyxia, froth at mouth.<br>• Haemorrhagic areas at serosa surface, organs are congested.<br>• Spinal cord is congested. |

| Medico-legal aspects | • Accidental poisoning, strychnine intake is considered as aphrodisiac.<br>• Rarely homicide, used to kill cattles. |
|---|---|
| Therapeutic dose | • Less than 30 mg. |

Image 9.5 Seeds of Kupeelu

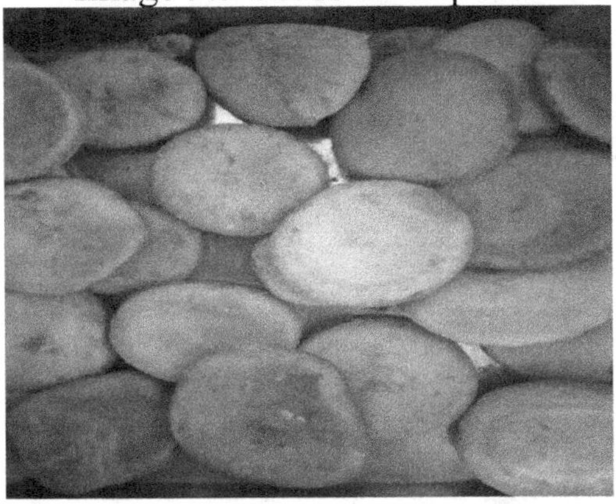

- **Ahiphena:**
  - **Botanical name**: Papaver somniferum
  - **Family**: Papaveraceae
  - **Kula**: Ahiphena Kula
  - **Type**: Neurotoxic poison
  - **Synonyms**: Aphima, Aphika, Nagaphena
  - **Toxic parts**: Seeds
  - **Toxic principles**: Morphine, codeine, papaverine.
  - **Mechanism of action**: Cocaine is CNS stimulant.
  - Absorption from oral, nasal and respiratory sites.
  - Metabolism is in liver and excretion through urine.
  - **Fatal dose**: Crude opium: 1-2gm, tincture opium : 3-4ml, morphine: 60-180mg, heroine: 20-30mg.
  - **Fatal period**: 45 minutes to 12 hours.

Table 9.7

| | |
|---|---|
| **Signs and symptoms** | a) stage of excitement: Stage of well being and increased mental and physical activities. Freedom from anxiety. Hallucination. Flushing of face.<br>b) stage of stupor: Headache, fatigue, giddiness, heaviness of body.<br>c) stage of coma |
| **Management** | • Juice extracted from the plant of Bruhatkshudra in 1 Pala quantity.<br>• Covering the patient for maintaining body heat. Rubbing palm and soles for warmth.<br>• Naloxane: 0.4-2gm, Nalorphine: 5-10gm |
| **Post-mortem appearance** | • Injection marks, cyanosis, white froth around mouth and nose, petechiae. |
| **Medico-legal aspects** | • Homicidal poison and accidental poison in children. |
| **Therapeutic dose** | • Purified resin: 30-125mg, powder: 1-2gm, seeds: 2-5gm |

Image of 9.6 Flower of Ahiphena

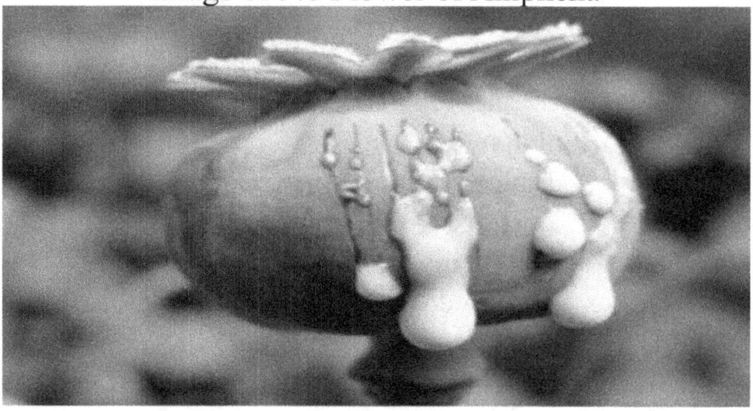

- **Dhattura:**
    - **Botanical name**: Dhatura alba
    - **Family**: Solanaceae
    - **Kula**: Kantakari Kula
    - **Type**: Neurotoxic poison

- **Synonyms**: Dhatura, Kanaka, Shivapriya, Mahamohi, Kanakahvya, Kantaphala, Ghantapushpa.
- **Toxic parts**: Seeds and flowers
- **Toxic principles**: Scopolamine, Hyoscyamine, Atropine.
- **Fatal dose**: 50-100 seeds, 10-100mg morphine.
- **Fatal period**: 2 hours

Table 9.8

| | |
|---|---|
| **Signs and symptoms** | • 9D: Dry hot skin, dilatation of cutaneous blood vessels, dilatation of pupils, dryness of throat and mouth, delirium, drowsiness, drunken gait, dysphagia, difficulty in talking. |
| **Management** | • Treat in quiet and dark environment.<br>• Gastric lavage, catheterization of bladder.<br>• Purgatives because intestinal motility is decreased.<br>• Monitor and regulate the temperature.<br>• Agitation can be controlled by judicious use of diazepam.<br>• Hyperpyrexia treated by hydration and cold sponging.<br>• Antidote: Physostigmine given slowly over 5-10 minutes. |
| **Post-mortem appearance** | • Dilated pupils, seeds don't get putrefied and so can be found after death. |
| **Medico-legal aspects** | • Accidental intake of Dhattura seeds as chilli seeds.<br>• Suicidal poisoning, homicidal poisoning.<br>• Criminal responsibility: Seeds induce temporary insanity.<br>• Scopolamine used as a truth serum. |
| **Therapeutic dose** | • Seeds after purification: 50-100mg, root powder: 62.5-250mg. |

Image 9.7 Thorny seed holder of Dhattura

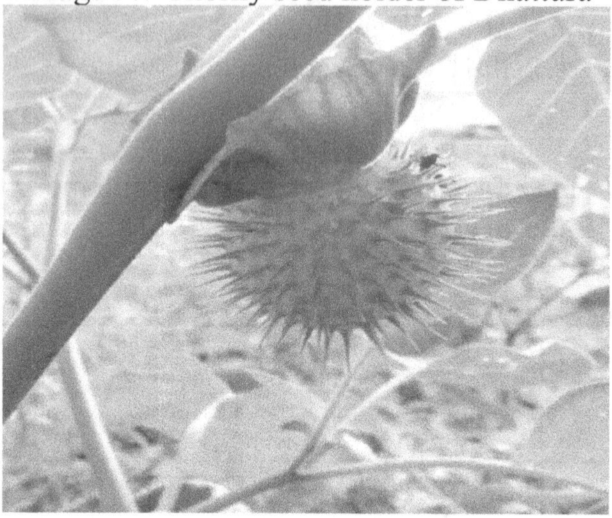

- **Bhanga:**
  - **Botanical name**: Cannabis sativa
  - **Family**: Cannabaceae
  - **Kula**: Bhanga Kula
  - **Type**: Neurotoxic poison
  - **Synonyms**: Marijuana
  - **Toxic parts**: Leaves
  - **Toxic principles**: Cannabinol, Cannabidinol, Cannabichromene
  - **Mechanism of action**: GIT and respiratory tract, subcutaneous and IM injection.
  - Metabolism is in liver.
  - Excretion through bile, urine, faeces.
  - **Fatal dose**: Charas: 2 gm/kg, Ganja: 8 gm/kg, Bhanga: 10 gm/kg.
  - **Fatal period**: 12 hours.

Table 9.9

| | |
|---|---|
| **Signs and symptoms** | • Symptoms of multiple sclerosis, sedative and analgesic. Now it is a banned drug all over the world. |
| **Management** | • Gut decontamination, benzodiazepine for paranoia.<br>• Haloperidol for acute psychotic state.<br>• Supportive measures. |
| **Post-mortem appearance** | • Signs of asphyxia, unabsorbed Bhanga may be identified in stomach. |
| **Medico-legal aspects** | • Drug of abuse, acute intoxication causes impairment in motor skills and judgment.<br>• Induces suicidal ideation, homicidal poisoning. |
| **Therapeutic dose** | • Leaf powder: 125-250mg, Ganja: 60-125mg, Charas: 30mg in divided doses in a day. |

Image 9.8 Plant of Bhanga

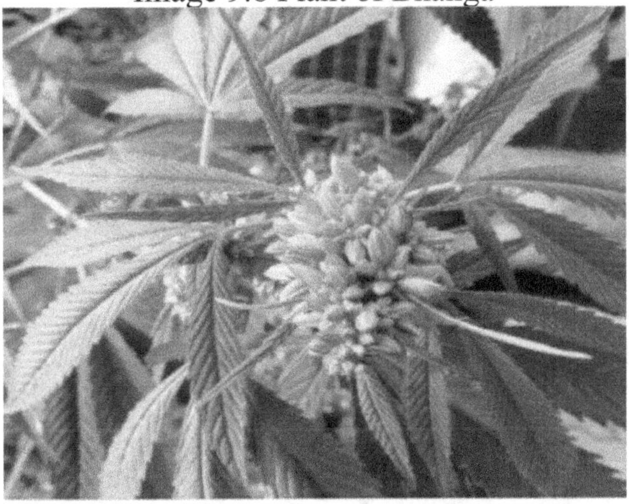

### 3. Irritant poisons:

- ***Jayapala:***
  - **Botanical name**: Croton tiglium
  - **Family**: Euphorbiaceae
  - **Kula**: Eranda Kula
  - **Type**: Irritant poison
  - **Synonyms**: Rechaka, Beeja rechaka, Danti beeja,

Maladravi, Sheegra, Nikumba, Chitramoola.

- **Toxic parts**: Seed, stem, leaves.
- **Toxic principles**: Crotin, Crotonoside, Crotonoleic acid, Crotonol.
- **Mechanism of action**: Toxalbumin in seeds is a toxic protein which disables ribosomes and disrupts protein synthesis.
- **Fatal dose**: 20 drops of oil in adults, 1 seed or 3 drops of oil in children.
- **Fatal period**: 4-6 hours.

Table 9.10

| | |
|---|---|
| **Signs and symptoms** | • Pain in abdomen, salivation, vomiting, diarrhoea.<br>• Vertigo, circulatory failure, shock. |
| **Management** | • Gastric lavage, fluid and electrolyte balance, symptomatic treatment. |
| **Post-mortem appearance** | • Signs of inflammation in GIT, gastric mucosa congested. |
| **Medico-legal aspects** | • Accidental poisoning, procure abortion.<br>• Seeds used in homicidal poisoning.<br>• Used in quack medicine.<br>• Arrow poisoning. |
| **Therapeutic dose** | • Seed: 25-50mg, seed oil: 1-2 drops. |

Image 9.9 Plant of Jayapala

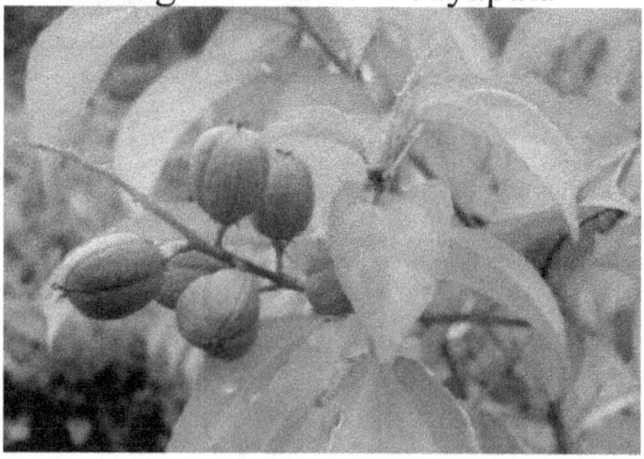

- **Gunja:**
    - Botanical name: Abrus precatorius
    - Family: Fabaceae
    - Kula: Shimbi Kula
    - Type: Irritant poison
    - Synonyms: Chudamani, Kakanatika, Kakasahvaya, Shikhandika, Sheetapaki, Krushnala, Raktika, Vanavasini, Kakachincha.
    - Toxic parts: Seed, root, leaves.
    - Toxic principles: Abrin, similar to viper snake venom.
    - Fatal dose: 1-2 crushed seeds, 90-120mg abrin
    - Fatal period: 3-5 days

Table 9.11

| | |
|---|---|
| **Signs and symptoms** | • Painful swelling, ecchymosis, necrosis.<br>• Nausea, vomiting, bloody diarrhoea, abdominal pain. |
| **Management** | • Antidote: Anti-abrin be provided.<br>• HCL+Pepsin.<br>• Sodium bicarbonate to maintain alkalinity of urine.<br>• Symptomatic treatment. |
| **Post-mortem appearance** | • Congestion of GIT, local oedema-inflammation-necrosis.<br>• Cerebral oedema, liver-spleen-kidney congestion.<br>• The symptoms resemble to viper snake bite. |
| **Medico-legal aspects** | • Accidental poisoning, homicidal poisoning, cattle poisoning<br>• Malingerers use abrin powder to procure conjunctivitis.<br>• Intact seeds, boiled seeds, cooked seeds when ingested are not poisonous. |
| **Therapeutic dose** | • Used externally only. |

Image 9.10 Plant and seeds of Gunja

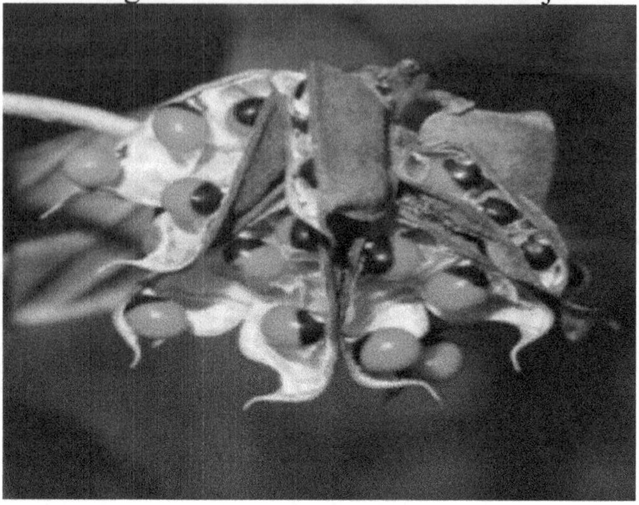

- **Bhallataka:**
    - **Botanical name**: Semecarpus anacardium
    - **Family**: Anacardaceae
    - **Kula**: Amra Kula
    - **Type**: Irritant poison
    - **Synonyms**: Bilava, Tapana, Dahana, Arushkara, Shophakara, Vrankruta, Taila beeja.
    - **Toxic parts**: Nut
    - **Toxic principles**: Semecarpol, bhilawanol, bioflavonoids, anacardic acid.
    - **Fatal dose**: 5-8 seeds, 10 gm of marking nut.
    - **Fatal period**: 12-24 hours.

Table 9.12

| | |
|---|---|
| **Signs and symptoms** | • Dermal: irritation, inflammation, vesication, blisters, pain, itching, ulcers with sloughing of skin.<br>• Ingestion: blister in oral cavity, vomiting, diarrhoea, hypotension, delirium, shock, coma. |
| **Management** | • Gastric lavage, milk, coconut water, supportive measures. |

| Post-mortem appearance | • Blister formation in and around oral cavity, throat, GI inflammation.<br>• Fatty degeneration of liver has been found. |
|---|---|
| Medico-legal aspects | • Accidental poisoning in quack medicine.<br>• Juice applied on external genitalia of female as a punishment for infidelity.<br>• Used to fabricate wound, juice thrown to cause injury.<br>• Juice applied over the cervical OS to procure criminal abortion.<br>• Skin lesion produced by marking nut may be confused with contusion. |
| Therapeutic dose | • Taila: 12-20 drops, Ksheerapaka: 30 ml. |

Image 9.11 Plant of Bhallataka

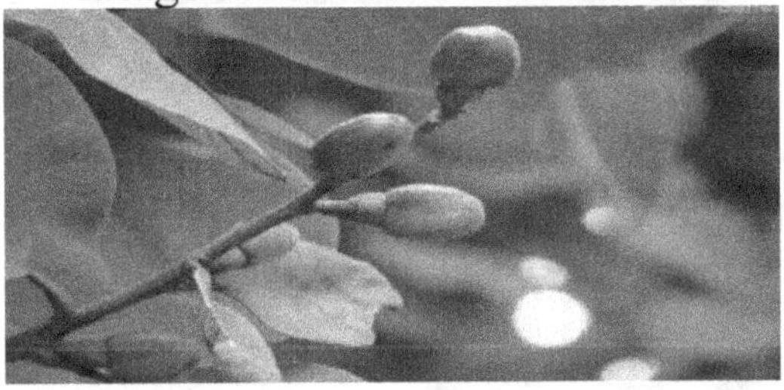

- **Arka:**
    - **Botanical name**: Calotropis procera
    - **Family**: Apocynacaea
    - **Kula**: Arka Kula
    - **Type**: Irritant poison
    - **Synonyms**: Toolaphala, Ksheeraparna, Arkaparna, Vikirana, Asphota, Raktapushpa, Sapushpa, Talaphala.
    - **Toxic parts**: Root, stem, leaves. Roots being more poisonous.
    - **Toxic principles**: Calotropin, Calatoxin, Uscharin, Calactin.
    - **Fatal dose**: Latex: 500mg
    - **Fatal period**: 30 minutes- 8 hours

Table 9.13

| | |
|---|---|
| **Signs and symptoms** | • Diarrhoea, vomiting, skin allergy.<br>• Latex going in eye causes blindness due to corneal opacity, pupil dilatation.<br>• Excessive salivation, stomatitis, tetanic convulsions, delirium. |
| **Management** | • External: Chinchapatra Kalka application, sunlight.<br>• Internal: Goghrita or Palasha as antidote, Gairik siddha jala.<br>• Gastric lavage, activated charcoal, morphine to relieve pain, diazepam for convulsions, maintain vitals.<br>• In dermal exposure wash the affected area with water. |
| **Post-mortem appearance** | • Signs of irritation in stomach and intestine.<br>• Bloody discharge from nostrils, frothy mouth, empty heart, spleen-kidney-liver congested. |
| **Medico-legal aspects** | • Criminal abortion, infanticide, homicide.<br>• Accidental poisoning, cattle poison, artificial wound formation. |
| **Therapeutic dose** | • Root bark powder: 0.5-1gm, flower powder: 1-2gm. |

Image 9.12 Plant of Arka

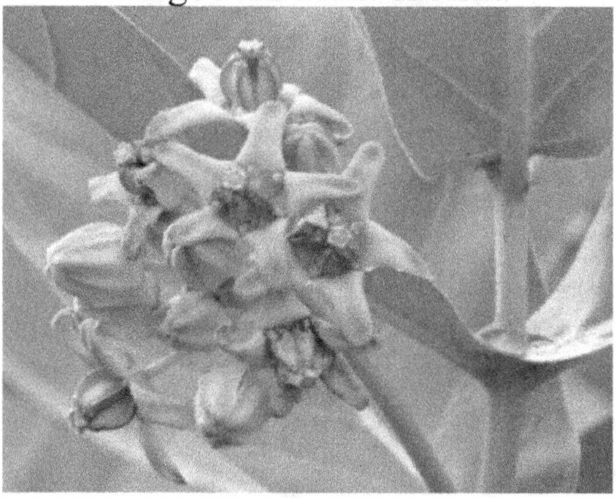

- **Snuhi:**
  - Botanical name: Euphorbia neriifolia
  - Family: Euphorbiaceae

- Kula: Eranda Kula
- Type: Irritant poison
- Synonyms: Sudha, Samantha dugdha, Nistrisha patra, Bahushaka, Ksheerakanda, Vatari, Vajradruma.
- Toxic parts: Latex of stem and leaves.
- Toxic principles: Euphorbol, euphol, tulipanin.
- Mechanism of action: Irritant organic vegetative poison.
- Fatal dose: 25-30 ml
- Fatal period: 3 days

Table 9.14

| | |
|---|---|
| **Signs and symptoms** | • Skin burning sensation, swelling.<br>• Eye contact causes burning sensation and swelling.<br>• Diarrhoea, vomiting, unconsciousness. |
| **Management** | • External: Chinchapatra Kalka application, sunlight.<br>• Internal: Goghrita or milk as antidote, Gairik siddha jala.<br>• Wash area under running water, gastric lavage.<br>• Skin irritation: topical corticosteroids.<br>• Eye irritation: antibiotic eyedrops. |
| **Post-mortem appearance** | • Signs of inflammation in contact part, gangrene patches in stomach, rotten spleen. |
| **Medico-legal aspects** | • Accidental poisoning, suicidal poisoning, homicidal poisoning.<br>• Criminal abortion. |
| **Therapeutic dose** | • Root powder: 0.5-1gm, stem juice: 5-10ml, milky latex: 125-250 mg. |

Image 9.13 Plant of Snuhi

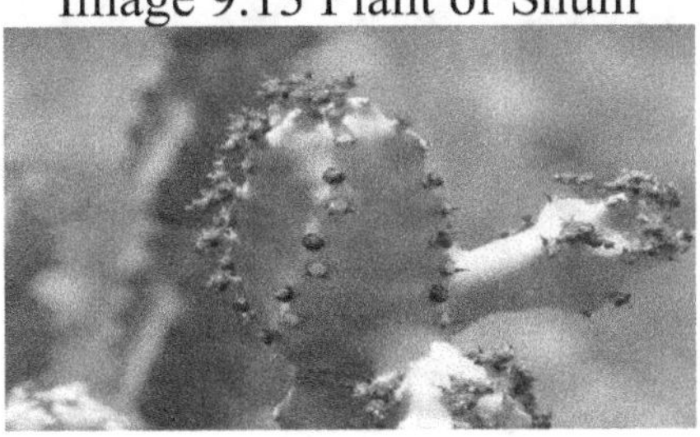

- **Langali:**
    - **Botanical name**: Gloriosa superba
    - **Family**: Liliaceae
    - **Kula**: Rasona Kula
    - **Type**: Irritant poison
    - **Synonyms**: Raktapushpa, Agnishika, Shukrapushpi, Halini, Indrapushpi, Garbhapatini.
    - **Toxic parts**: Rhizome, tuber.
    - **Toxic principles**: Colchicine, puteolin, colchicamide.
    - **Fatal dose**: Abortifacient: 3-6gm, powder: 2-5gm, colchicine: 7-60mg.
    - **Fatal period**: 12-72 hours

Table 9.15

| | |
|---|---|
| **Signs and symptoms** | • Burning and numb mouth, nausea, vomiting, convulsion, purgation, sweating. |
| **Management** | • Common treatment, symptomatic treatment, maintain blood pressure. |
| **Post-mortem appearance** | • Not specific |
| **Medico-legal aspects** | • Accidental poisoning as tuber is mistaken for sweet potato.<br>• Suicidal poisoning, abortifacient. |
| **Therapeutic dose** | • 250 to 500mg |

Image 9.14 Plant of Langali

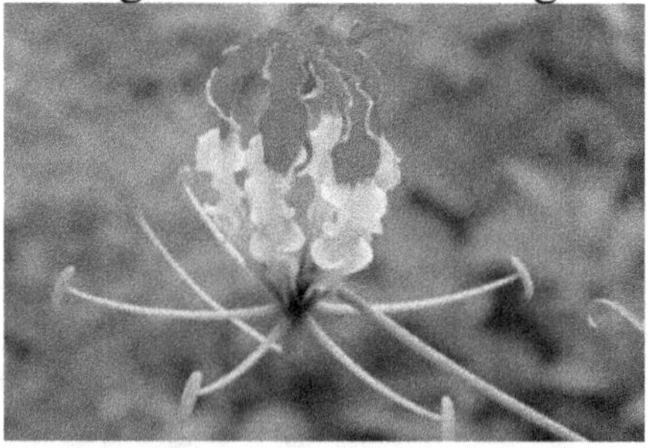

**Multiple Choice Questions:**

**1. What is the botanical name of Gunja?**
A. Calotropis procera B. Semecarpus anacardium
C. Abrus precatorius D. Euphorbia neriifolia

**2. What is the Kula of Snuhi?**
A. Eranda B. Rasona C. Arka D. Amra

**3. What is the fatal dose for the extract of Vatsanabha?**
A. 1-2gm B. 25 drops C. 250mg D. 4mg

**4. What is the therapeutic dose of purified resin of Ahiphena?**
A. 10-20mg B. 30-125mg C. 200mg D. 175mg

**5. Vishamooshika is the synonym of?**
A. Langali B. Hrutpatti C. Kupeelu D. Bhanga

**6. Fox glove is the synonym of?**
A. Karveera B. Vatsanabha C. Dhattura D. Hrutpatti

**7. What is the toxic part of Cerebra odollam?**
A. Fruits B. Leaves C. Roots D. Stem

**8. Which of the following is not a neurotoxic poison?**
A. Kupeelu B. Ahiphena C. Bhanga D. Snuhi

**9. Which of the following is an irritant poison?**
A. Vatsanabha B. Jayapala C. Karveera D. Tobacco

**10. Vatsanabha belongs to which family?**
A. Euphorbiaceae B. Apocynaceae
C. Ranunculaceae D. Anacardaceae

**11. What is not a toxic principle in Karveera?**
A. Oleandrin B. Neriin C. Cerberia D. Brucine

**12. Scopolamine is a toxic principle found in?**
A. Langali B. Dhattura C. Karveera D. Jayapala

**13. What is the Kula of Langali?**
A. Rasona B. Eranda C. Arka D. Amra

**14. What is the therapeutic dose of Bhallatak Ksheeraoaka?**
A. 10ml B. 30ml C. 20ml D. 40ml

**15. Toolaphala is the synonym of?**
A. Langali B. Vatsanabha C. Arka D. Karveera

**Answer key for MCQs:**

| | |
|---|---|
| 1 | C |
| 2 | A |
| 3 | C |
| 4 | B |
| 5 | C |
| 6 | D |
| 7 | A |
| 8 | D |

| | |
|---|---|
| 9 | B |
| 10 | C |
| 11 | D |
| 12 | B |
| 13 | A |
| 14 | B |
| 15 | C |

# Ch. 10

# Sthavara Visha: Poisons of Metallic Origin

**1. Arsenic poisoning:**

- **Properties**: Arsenic is a metalloid and not very toxic. Arsenic salts are more toxic.
- **Sources**: Rocks and soil, drinking water, sea water, fruits and vegetables, sea foods, industrial source.
- **Uses**: Rodenticides, in alloys, colouring agent.
- **Absorption**: Skin, inhalation, GIT mucosa, cutaneous absorption.
- **Metabolism**: Liver, kidney.
- **Excretion**: Urine.
- **Mechanism of action**:
    - o Arsenic blocks Krebs cycle and interrupts oxidative phosphorylation causing depletion of ATP and cell death occurs.
    - o Inhibits transformation of thiamine into acetyl CoA and Succinyl-CoA. This causes thiamine deficiency.
    - o Phosphorus in the bones get replaced.

Table 10.1

| | |
|---|---|
| **Signs and symptoms** | • Nausea, vomiting, diarrhoea, gastroenteritis, abdominal pain.<br>• Pigment changes, palmoplantar hyperkeratoses.<br>• Uraemia, tachycardia, vertigo, tremors, convulsions.<br>• Collapse and circulatory failure. |
| **Management** | • Stomach wash<br>• Antidote: Freshly precipitated hydrated ferric oxide. |

| Post-mortem appearance | • Red velvety stomach mucosa, sub-mucosal petechial haemorrhage.<br>• Fatty degeneration of kidney, heart, liver.<br>• Putrefied bones, hairs, nails. |
|---|---|

Image 10.1

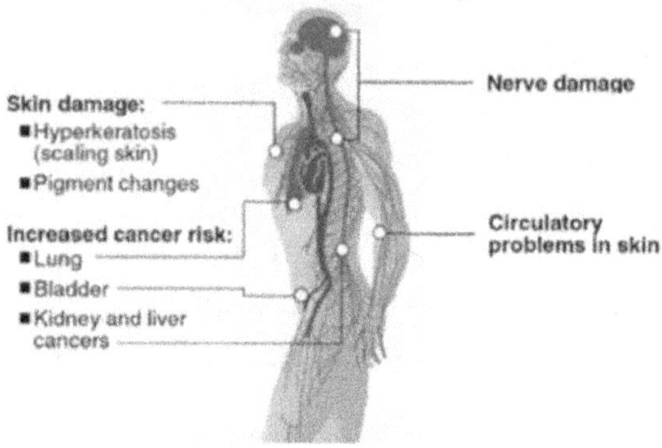


**2. Mercury poisoning:**

- **Properties:** It is an element found in air, water, soil. In-utero exposure or early childhood exposure can cause to growth retardation. Has toxic effects on nervous system, digestive system and immune system.
- **Sources:** Fish and shellfish contaminated with methylmercury. Batteries, thermometers, barometers, electrical switches, lamps, skin lightening products, cosmetics, pharmaceuticals.

Table 10.2

| Signs | • Paraesthesia, itching, burning pain, feeling of insects crawling on skin.<br>• Pink cheeks, fingertips and toes.<br>• Shedding and peeling of skin.<br>• Children show: red cheeks, swelling, loss of hairs, teeth, nails.<br>• Muscle weakness, photophobhia. |
|---|---|

| | |
|---|---|
| **Symptoms** | • Metallic taste in mouth, burning pain in mouth, tongue and throat corroded with white coating.<br>• Bloody red stool, nausea, vomiting.<br>• Headache, numbness, convulsions, tremors. |
| **Diagnosis** | • Physical findings, exposure to mercury.<br>• Blood test: elevated mercury levels. |
| **Treatment** | • Decontamination: Remove clothes, wash skin with soap and water, clean eyes with saline solution.<br>• Chelating agent: DMSA, DMPS, BAL and D-Penicillamine. |

Image 10.2

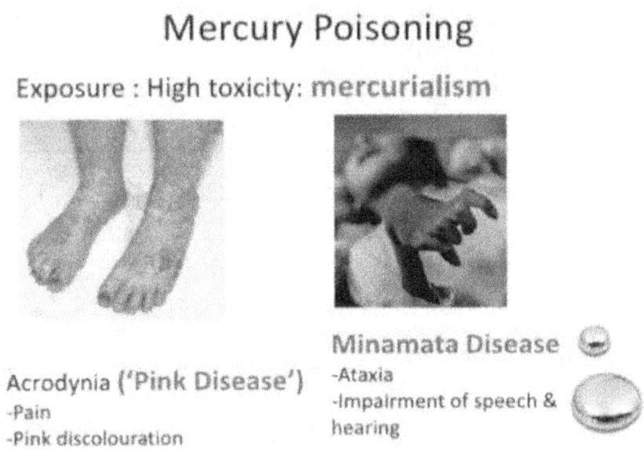


**3. Lead poisoning:**

- **Properties**: Mercury is a naturally occurring toxic metal in earth's crust. Extensive uses has shown bad effects on human health.
- **Sources**: Mining, smelting, manufacturing and recycling activities. Manufacturing of lead-acid batteries for motor vehicles. Pigments, paints, stained glass, jewellery, toys, traditional cosmetics like sindoor.

Table 10.3

| | |
|---|---|
| **Common Symptoms** | • Metallic taste in mouth, abdominal pain, vomiting, bloody red stool.<br>• Headache, drowsiness, cramps, numbness.<br>• Blue gum line in chronic poisoning. |
| **Symptoms in new born** | • Pre mature birth, low birth weight, slow growth, delayed milestone achievement, high blood pressure. |
| **Symptoms in children** | • Learning difficulties, irritability, loss of appetite, weight loss, sluggishness, fatigue.<br>• Abdominal pain, constipation, vomiting, hearing loss, PICA. |
| **Symptoms in adults** | • Memory decrease, difficulty in concentration, headache, abdominal pain.<br>• Mood disorders, decreased sperm count, miscarriage, abortions. |
| **Diagnosis** | • Metallic taste, blood levels show high lead. |
| **Treatment** | • Plenty of warm water, milk, egg white, barley water.<br>• Induce vomiting, chelating agent: EDTA.<br>• Antidote: DMSA. |

Image 10.3

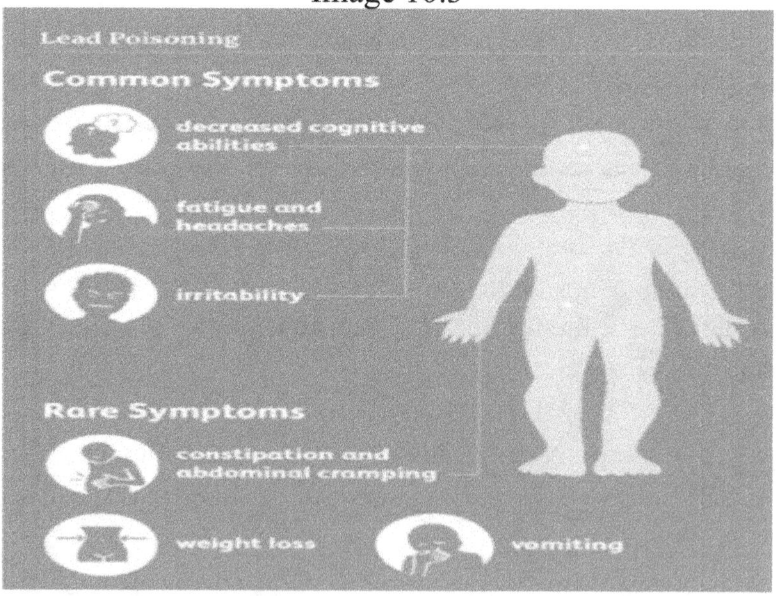

**4. Copper poisoning**

- **Properties**: pure copper is not poisonous but copper salts are poisonous. Anhydrous $CuSO4$ has grey-white colour and pentahydrate has bright blue colour.
- **Sources**: Insecticide, fungicide, alloys and pigments.
- **Absorption**: Skin, mucous membrane, inhalation, GIT.
- **Excretion**: Saliva, bile, milk.

Table 10.4

| | |
|---|---|
| **Acute poisoning signs and symptoms** | 1. Ingestion:<br>• Metallic taste, increased salivation, colicky abdominal pain, diarrhoea, nausea.<br>• Vomiting with bluish greenish vomitus.<br>• Oliguria, renal failure.<br>• Convulsions, delirium, coma.<br>2. Inhalation of copper fuels:<br>• Respiratory tract irritation, cough, conjunctivitis. |
| **Chronic poisoning signs and symptoms** | • Abdominal pain, greenish lines on gum margins.<br>• Vineyard sprayer's lung disease: interstitial pulmonary lesions leading to respiratory insufficiency.<br>• Greenish discoloration of hair,<br>• Wilson disease: build up of copper in liver, brain, eyes. Kayser-Fleischer rings. |
| **Treatment** | • Gastric lavage with potassium ferrocyanide.<br>• Chelation therapy: Dimercaprol 2.5 mg/kg 4 hourly IM followed by oral penicillamine 2gm/day.<br>• Symptomatic treatment. |
| **Post-mortem appearance** | • Greenish blue froth at mouth, blue lines on gums, greenish blue gastric mucosa and stomach contents.<br>• Haemolysis, kidney tubular necrosis, eosinophilic cast appearance, oedema in medulla.<br>• Liver microscopy shows centri-lobular necrosis. |
| **Medico-legal aspects** | • Accidental poisoning, suicidal poisoning.<br>• Chronic poisoning: industrial hazard.<br>• Used to procure abortion, cattle poisoning. |

Image 10.4

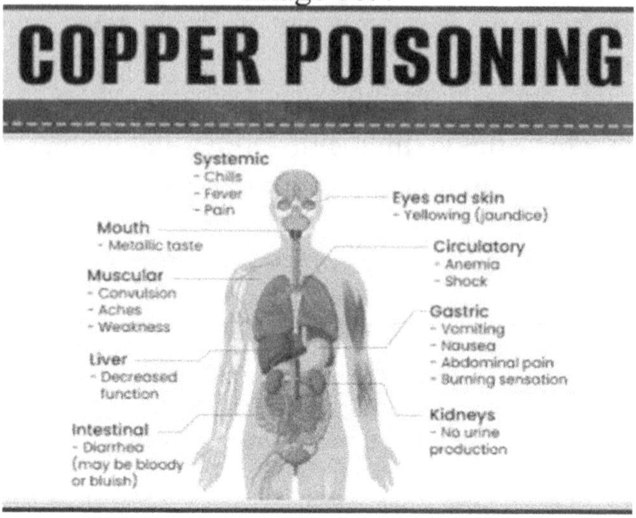


**Multiple Choice Questions:**

**1. Pink disease is found in which metal poisoning?**

A. Copper B. Lead C. Arsenic D. Mercury

**2. Greenish blue froth at mouth found in which poisoning?**

A. Lead B. Copper C. Mercury D. Arsenic

**3. Lead poisoning antidote is which of the following?**

A. DMSA B. DMPS C. D-Penicillamine D. BAL

**4. Paraesthesia is a symptom of which poisoning?**

A. Copper B. Lead C. Arsenic D. Mercury

**5. Blue gum line is symptom of which chronic poisoning?**

A. Mercury B. Arsenic C. Lead D. Copper

**6. Which metal blocks Krebs cycle and interrupts oxidative phosphorylation?**

A. Copper B. Arsenic C. Mercury D. Lead

**7. Palmoplantar hyperkeratoses is a symptom of which poisoning?**

A. Lead B. Mercury C. Arsenic D. Copper

**8. Kayser-Fleischer ring is found in which poisoning?**

A. Copper B. Arsenic C. Lead D. Mercury

**9. Minimata disease found in which metal poisoning?**

A. Lead B. Arsenic C. Mercury D. Copper

**10. D-Penicillamine is a chelating agent for which metallic poisoning treatment?**

A. Copper B. Lead C. Arsenic D. Mercury

**Answer key for MCQs:**

| | |
|---|---|
| 1 | D |
| 2 | B |
| 3 | A |
| 4 | D |
| 5 | C |

| | |
|---|---|
| 6 | B |
| 7 | C |
| 8 | A |
| 9 | C |
| 10 | D |

# Ch. 11
# Jangama Visha

**Jangama Visha:**

सर्पाः कीटोन्दुरा लूता वृश्चिका गृहगोधिकाः।
जलौकामत्स्यमण्डूकाः कणभाः सकृकण्टकाः।।
श्वसिंहव्याघ्रगोमायुतरक्षुनकुलादयः।
दंष्ट्रिणो ये विषं तेषां दंष्ट्रोत्थं जङ्गमं मतम्।।
(च.चि.२३/६–१०)

Jangama Visha are Sarpa (snakes), Keeta (insects), Luta (spiders), Vrushchika (scorpion), Gruha godhika (house lizards), Jalauka (leeches), Matsya (fishes), Manduka (frogs), Kanabha (locusts), Krukantaka (chameleons), Shwa (dogs), Simha (lions), Vyaghra (tigers), Gomayu (jackal), Takashu (hyena), Nakula (mongoose) are the animals having fangs. These cause poisoning.

**Jangama Visha Samanya Lakshana:**

निद्रां तन्द्रां क्लमं दाहं सपाकं लोमहर्षणम्।
शोफं चैवातिसारं च जनयेज्जङ्गमं विषम।। (च.चि.२३/१५)

Sleeping, laziness, exertion without working (mental fatigue), burning sensation, suppuration, horripilation, swelling, diarrhoea.

**1. Sarpa Visha:**

Image 11.1

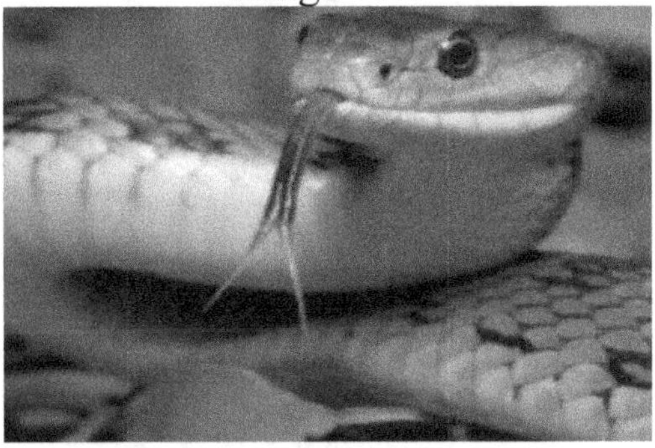

- ***Sarpa Bheda (Types of snakes)***
  - There are more than 2000 species of snakes in the world and approximately 217 species in India.
  - According to Acharya Charak: Mandali, Rajimana.

Table 11.1 Types of snake according to Acharya Sushruta

| Names | Numbers |
|---|---|
| Darvikara | 26 |
| Mandali | 22 |
| Nirvisha | 12 |
| Rajimaha | 10 |
| Vaikaranja & Vaikaranjaudabhava | 10 |

Table 11.2 Types of snake according to Acharya Vagbhata

| Divine snakes | Terrestrial snakes |
|---|---|
| 1 Ananta | Darvikara |
| 2 Takshaka | Mandali |
| 3 Vasuki | Nirvisha |
| 4 Gulika | Rajimana |
| 5 Katkotaka | Vyantara |
| 6 Shamkhapala | |
| 7 Padma | |
| 8 Maha-padma | |

- **Sarpa bheda and it's effects on Dosha:**

  इह दर्वीकरः सर्पो मण्डली राजिमानिति।
  त्रयो यथाक्रमं वातपित्तश्लेष्मप्रकोपणाः।। (च.चि.२३/१२४)

Darvikara Sarpa aggravate Vayu, Mandali Sarpa aggravate Pitta, Rajimana Sarpa aggravate Kapha.

- **Types of Sarpa based on Linga bheda:** Purusha, Stree, Napunsaka.

- **Types of Sarpa based on Varna bheda:**

Table 11.3

| | |
|---|---|
| ब्राह्मण | मुक्तारुप्यप्रभा, कपिल, पन्नगा, सुंगधय, सुवर्णामारुते. |
| क्षत्रिय | स्निग्धवर्णा, पन्नगा, भृशकोपना, सूर्यचंद्राकृति, छन्नलक्ष्य, पारावतामा. |
| वैश्य | कृष्णा, वज्रनिभा, लोहिता, पारावतामा. |
| शुद्र | महिष, दीपिकावर्ग, परुष, भिन्नवर्णा |

- **Sarpa parichaya:**

  दर्वीकरः फणी ज्ञेयो मण्डली मण्डलाफणः।
  बिन्दुलेखविचित्राङ्गः पन्नगः स्यात्तु राजिमान।।
  (च.चि.२३/१२५)

Table 11.4 Identification of snakes

| | |
|---|---|
| Darvikara Sarpa | Phani (hood) |
| Mandali Sarpa | Aphana (hoodless) but has Mandalas |
| Rajimana Sarpa | Bindu Lekha Vichitranga (streaks on body) |

- सर्पदंश कारण (**Reasons and kinds of bite**):

  पादाभिमृष्टा दुष्टा वा क्रुद्धा ग्रासार्थिनोऽपि वा।
  ते दशन्ति महाक्रोधास्त्रिविधं भीमदर्शनाः।।
  सर्पितं रदितं चापि तृतीयमथ निर्विषम्।

सर्पाङ्गाभिहतं केचिदिच्छन्ति खलु तद्विदः।। (सु.क.४/१३)

When snakes are tread on, snakes which are angry in nature, who are in search of food bite humans. Their bite can be Sarpita, Radita and Nirvisha type. Some also include Sarpangabhihata.

- सर्पदंश लक्षण (**Features of snake bite**):

पदानि यत्र दन्तानामेकं द्वे वा बहूनि वा।
निमग्नान्यल्परक्तानि यान्युद्वृत्य करोति हि।।
चञ्चुमालकयुक्तानि वैकृत्यकरणानि च।
सङ्क्षिप्तानि सशोफानि विद्यात्तत् सर्पितं भिषक।।
(सु.क.४/१५–१६)

Two or more bite marks seen at the site of bite, minute amount of blood coming out of site, when squeezed eruptions are seen, swelling present are symptoms to be understood as poisonous bite.

- रदित दंश लक्षण (**Laccrated bite features**):

राज्यः सलोहिता यत्र नीलाः पीताः सितास्तथा।
विज्ञेयं रदितं तत्तु ज्ञेयमल्पविषं च तत्।। (सु.क.४/१७)

Bluish-red, yellow, white bite lines are present are Radita (laccrated) bites. These are less poisonous in nature.

- निर्विष दंश लक्षण (Poison free bite)

अशोफमल्पदुष्टासृक् प्रकृतिस्थस्य देहिनः।
पदं पदानि वा विद्यादविषं तच्चिकित्सकः।।
सर्पस्पृष्टस्य भीरोर्हि भयेन कुपितोऽनिलः।
कस्यचित् कुरुते शोफं सर्पाङ्गाभिहतं तु तत्।।
(सु.क.४/१८–१९)

No swelling, little amount of vitiated blood, snake is not angry, one or more visible bite marks at site be understood as Nirvisha (non-poisonous) bite. In some persons, there occurs swelling at touch site due to Vata aggravation, this is called as Sarpangabhihata.

- **Sarpa Visha Visheshata:**

विशेषाद्रूक्षकटुकमम्लोष्णं स्वादु शीतलम्।
विषं यथाक्रमं तेषां तस्माद्वातादिकोपनम।। (च.चि.२३/१२६)

Table 11.5 Properties of snake bite

| Sarpa | Properties | Aggravated Dosha |
|---|---|---|
| Darvikara Sarpa | Ruksha, Katu | Vata |
| Mandali Sarpa | Amla, Ushna | Pitta |
| Rajimana Sarpa | Madhura, Sheeta | Kapha |

- **Sarpa Visha Samanya Lakshana:**

विषं हि निशितनिस्त्रिंशाशनिहुतवहदेश्यमाशुकारि
मुहर्तमप्युपेक्षितमातुरमतिपातयति....। (सु.क.४/३६)

Poison is similar to a sharp sword, lightening and fire. Kills the person in a Muhurta (48 minutes).

- **Sarpa Visha Vishesha Lakshana:**

***A. Darvikara Sarpa:***

दर्वीकरकृतो दंशः सूक्ष्मदंष्ट्रापदोऽसितः।
निरुद्धरक्तः कूर्माभो वातव्याधिकरो मतः।। (च.चि.२३/१२७)

Table 11.6 Features of Darvikara Sarpa bite

| | |
|---|---|
| Sukshma Samshtra | Minute fang marks |
| Krishna Varna | Black |
| Niruddha Rakta | Absence of bleeding |
| Kurmabho | Swelling resembles the shape of back of tortoise |
| Vata Vyadhikara | Diseases due to Vata Dosha occurs |

### *B. Mandali Sarpa:*

पृथ्वर्पितः सशोथश्च दंशो मण्डलिना कृतः।
पीताभः पीतरक्तश्च सर्वपित्तविकारकृत्।। (च.चि.२३/१२८)

Table 11.7 Features of Mandali Sarpa bite

| Pruthvarpita Sashotha | Swelling deep associated with swelling |
|---|---|
| Peeta | Yellowish discoloration at the site of bite |
| Pittarakta | Exudates at site of bite are yellow and bloody |
| Sarpa Pitta Vikaranuta | Diseases due to Pitta Dosha occurs |

### *C. Rajimana Sarpa:*

कृतो राजिमता दंशः पिच्छिलः स्थिरशोफकृत।
स्निग्धः पाण्डुश्च सान्द्रासृक् श्लेष्मव्याधिसमीरणः।।
(च.चि.२३/१२६)

Table 11.8 Features of Rajimana Sarpa bite

| Pichhila Sthira Shopha | Soft and stable oedema |
|---|---|
| Snigdha Pandu | Bite site is unctuous and pale |
| Sandra Asruka | Thick bloody exudate from site of bite |
| Shleshma Vyadhi | Diseases due to Kapha Dosha occurs |

- **Stree, Purusha, Kliba Sarpa:**

वृत्तभोगो महाकायः श्वसन्नूर्ध्वेक्षणः पुमान्।
स्थूलमूर्धा समाङ्गश्च स्त्री त्वतः स्याद्विपर्ययात्।।
क्लीबस्त्रसत्यधोदृष्टिः स्वरहीनः प्रकम्पते। (च.चि.२३/१३०)

Napumsaka Sarpa are fearful in nature.

Table 11.9 Difference between Stree, Purusha, Kliba Sarpa

| **Purusha** | **Stree** |
|---|---|
| Round coiled | No round coils |
| Large body | Small body |
| Hisses loudly | Doesn't hiss loudly |
| Looks upward | Doesn't look upward |
| Large head | Small head |

- **Sarpa Visha Vega Lakshana:**

Table 11.10

| Vega | Darvikara Damsha | Mandali Damsha | Rajimana Damsha |
|---|---|---|---|
| 1st | Blood becomes vitiated and black. This causes black complexion. Person feels as ant running on body. | Spreads into Rakta Dhatu causing yellowing. Oedema on bitten limb and burning sensation in whole body. | Spreads to Rakta Dhatu causing dull white discoloration, horripilation, person looks pale. |
| 2nd | Mamsa Dhatu gets vitiated causing swelling at bitten site. | Vitiates Mamsa Dhatu causing deep yellowing. Burning sensation all over body, oedema at bitten site. | Enters in Mamsa Dhatu, heaviness of body, fatigue, becomes more pale, oedema in the head. |
| 3rd | Medo Dhatu gets vitiated causes heaviness of head, vision loss, moistness at site of bite. | Medo Dhatu gets affected. Causes blurring of vision, intense thirst, putrefaction at the site, sweating. | Enters in Medo Dhatu. Causes blurring of vision, putrefaction at site, excess mucous secretion from nose, mouth, eyes. |
| 4th | Poison enters Koshtha causing excess salivation, vomiting, lethargy, joint pain. | Along with the above symptoms causes fever due to entry in Koshtha. | Spreads in Koshtha, heaviness of head, stiffness of neck |
| 5th | Poison enters Asthi Dhatu causing vitiation of Pranavayu and Agni. Causes joint pain, hiccups and burning sensation. | Burning sensation all over the body. | Dysphonia, dysarthria, fever. |
| 6th | Poison enters Majja Dhatu causes vitiation of Grahani. Sever pain in chest, heaviness in chest, delirium, diarrhoea. | Poison enters Majja Dhatu causes vitiation of Grahani. Sever pain in chest, heaviness in chest, delirium, diarrhoea. | Poison enters Majja Dhatu causes vitiation of Grahani. Sever pain in chest, heaviness in chest, delirium, diarrhoea. |
| 7th | Poison enters Shukra Dhatu causing excess phlegm from mouth, breaking pain in back and waist. Impaired functions of mind, body, suppression of breath leading to death. | Poison enters Shukra Dhatu causing excess phlegm from mouth, breaking pain in back and waist. Impaired functions of mind, body, suppression of breath leading to death. | Poison enters Shukra Dhatu causing excess phlegm from mouth, breaking pain in back and waist. Impaired functions of mind, body, suppression of breath leading to death. |

- **Sarpa Visha Samanya Chikitsa**

Table 11.11 General treatment for snake bites

| | | |
|---|---|---|
| Arishta Bandana | दंशस्योपरि बध्नीयादरिष्टां चतुरङ्गुले। क्षौमादिभिर्वेणिकया सिद्धैर्मन्त्रैश्च मन्त्रवित।। अम्बुवत् सेतुबन्धेन बन्धेन स्तभ्यते विषम। न वहन्ति सिराश्चास्य विषं बन्धाभिपीडिताः।। (अ.हृ.उ.३६/४२–४३) | Bandha be tied 4 Angula above site with rope, grass or cloth. Poison doesn't spread as blood vessels are subjected to pressure by binding. |
| Achushana, Chedana, Dahana | निष्पीड्यानूद्धेरद्दंशं मर्मसन्ध्यगतं तथा। न जायते विषाद्वेगो बीजनाशादिवाङ्कुरः।। (अ.हृ.उ.३६/४४) | Massage the site, remove fangs except for vital points. Stops further spread of poison. |
| Chetana Karma | दंशं मण्डलिनां मुक्त्वा पित्तलत्वादथापरम्। प्रतप्तैर्हेमलोहाद्यैर्दहेदाशूल्मुकेन वा।। करोति भस्मसात्सद्यो वह्निः किं नाम तु क्षतम् । (अ.हृ.उ.३६/४५–४६) | Except for Mandali snake bite having Pitta, other snake bite sites be burnt with heated rods of gold, iron or by burning charcoal. |
| Rakta Visraavana Kriya | विषे प्रविसृते विध्येत्सिरां सा परमा क्रिया।। रक्ते निर्ह्रियमाणे हि कृत्स्नं निर्ह्रीयते विषम्।। (अ.हृ.उ.३६/४८) | When poison has spread to the whole body, then cut the vein. This is the ultimate treatment as along with blood, poison also comes out. |

- Vamana Karma, Mani Prayoga, Agada Sevana, Aushadha Dharana, Sheetopachara can be done to treat the poisoning.

- **Sarpa Visha Veganusara Chikitsa:**

Table 11.12

| Vega | Darvikara Sarpa | Mandali Sarpa | Rajimana Sarpa |
|---|---|---|---|
| 1st | रक्तमोक्षण | रक्तमोक्षण | रक्तमोक्षण, घृतअगदपान |
| 2nd | मधु, घृत, अगदपान | मधु, घृत, अगदपान उपरान्त यवागू | वमन, अगदपान दर्वीकरवत् |
| 3rd | विषनाशक, नस्य, अन्जन | विरेचन, यवागूपान | दर्वीकरवत् |
| 4th | वमन, स्थावर विष प्रसंग वर्णित यवागू | दर्वीकरवत् | दर्वीकरवत् |
| 5th | शीतल उपचार, विरेचन, यवागू | दर्वीकरवत् | दर्वीकरवत् |
| 6th | शीतल उपचार, विरेचन, यवागू | काकोल्यादि, मधुरगण | तीक्ष्ण अंजन, |

| 7th | तीक्ष्ण अंजन, नस्य, तीक्ष्ण शस्त्रेण मूर्ध्नि काकपाद | अगदपान, अवपीडन नस्य | तीक्ष्ण अवपीडन नस्य, संज्ञास्थापन |
|---|---|---|---|
| विषघ्न योग | Sindhuvara root, Shveta, Girikarnika. | Manjishtha, Madhuyashti, Jivanti, Rishabhaka, Shveta, Kashmarya with leaf buds of Vata. | Powder of Trikatu, Ativisha, Kushtha, Grahadhooma, Harenuka, Tagara, Katuka with honey. |

- **Snakes:**

Snakes are classified into different families, genera and species based on their morphology and genetic features.

Table 11.13 Features of poisonous and non-poisonous snakes

| **Features** | **Poisonous snakes** | **Non poisonous snakes** |
|---|---|---|
| Belly scales | Large and covers the entire belly | Small or moderate sized but doesn't cover the entire belly |
| Head scales | • A pit between eye, nostril: pit viper<br>• Third labial touches eye and nasal shield: cobra or coral snake<br>• Central row of scales on the back enlarged and under the surface of mouth, has 4 infralabials with 4th being the largest: kraits | Small to moderate large in size |
| Fangs | Long and grooved | Short and solid |
| Tails | Compressed | Not compressed |
| Habits | Generally nocturnal | Generally not nocturnal |
| Bites | Two fang marks with or without marks of other teeth | A number of small marks in a row |

Table 11.14 Clinical features of snakes

| **Neurotoxic** | **Hemotoxic** | **Musculotoxic** |
|---|---|---|
| Minimal reaction locally with strong neurotoxicity. | Venoms having hemolysins and thromboplastin causing widespread endothelial damage and hemolysis. | Venom produces generalized muscle pain, weakness. |

| | | |
|---|---|---|
| Weakness of face and legs. | Severe oozing of blood at the site of bite. | Polymyositis, myoglobinuria |
| Paralysis of mouth initially followed by throat, respiratory muscles. | Coagulation abnormalities causing haemorrhagic shock. | Respiratory failure and renal failure. |
| Cobra venom causes convulsions and krait causes only paralysis. | Haematuria and haemoglobinuria. | Hypokalemia, increased enzymes. |
| Eg: Cobra, Coral cobra, Kraits. | Eg: Vipers. | Eg: Sea snakes. |

Table 11.15 Common Cobra signs and symptom, fatal dose, fatal period

| | |
|---|---|
| Signs and symptoms | • Immediate local pain, swelling, blisters and regional lymphadenopathy.<br>• Nausea, vomiting, contraction of frontalis muscle causing elevation of eyebrows.<br>• Ptosis, blurred vision, loss of vision due to mydriasis, peri-oral paraesthesia.<br>• Dysphasia, dysphagia, paralysis of palate and jaw muscles.<br>• Tongue paralysis, neck paralysis, respiratory arrest, chest tightness, shortness of breath.<br>• Profuse salivation, abdominal pain, blood pressure and heart rate abnormalities.<br>• Drowsiness, euphoria. |
| Fatal dose | -12 mg |
| Fatal period | -8 hours |

Table 11.16 King Cobra signs and symptoms, fatal dose, fatal period

| | |
|---|---|
| Signs and symptoms | Local effects: Pain, excessive swelling, necrosis<br>Systemic effects: Giddiness, ptosis, ophthalmoplegia, dysphagia, hypertension, bradycardia, respiratory failure, flaccid paralysis. |

| Fatal dose | 12-15 mg |
|---|---|
| Fatal period | 90 minutes – 24 hours |

Table 11.17 Russel's viper signs and symptoms, fatal dose, fatal period

| Signs and symptoms | • Area becomes red, swollen, painful with cellulitis.<br>• Continuous bleeding, blister formation, necrosis.<br>• Giddiness, abdominal pain, vomiting.<br>• Sweating, dilated pupils, no response to light.<br>• Hypotension, circulatory collapse, death. |
|---|---|
| Fatal dose | 12 mg |
| Fatal period | 4 days |

Table 11.18 Pit viper signs and symptoms, fatal dose, fatal period

| Signs and symptoms | • Severe local pain with swelling, bruises, trouble breathing, irregular heart rate.<br>• Minty metallic taste in mouth, numbness around mouth, tongue, feet, bite site.<br>• Swelling in lymph nodes around area of bite. |
|---|---|
| Fatal dose | 40 – 70 mg |
| Fatal period | 3 – 6 hours |

- **WHO snake bite management guidelines:**
    - Clean the wound with soap and potable water, apply sterilized dressing.
    - Reassurance
    - Pressure over the site of bite by using a tourniquet or cloth piece. This causes slow absorption of poison and occludes the venous and lymph drainage.
    - Limb immobilization.
    - Polyvalent Anti-snake Venom (PAV) be used within 4 hours of snake bite.
    - PAV each vial has 6-8 mg of neutralized snake venom. Approximately 10 vials be given.

- **Polyvalent Anti-snake Venom:**
    - Prepared by hyper-immunizing a horse against 4 common poisonous snakes: Cobra, Common krait, Russel's viper, Saw scaled viper.

**2. Loota Visha:**

लूताविषं घोरतमं दुर्विज्ञेयतमं च तत्।
दुश्चिकित्स्यतमं चापि भिषग्भिर्मन्दबुद्धिभिः।।
सविषं निर्विषं चौतदित्येवं परिशङ्किते।
विषघ्नमेव कर्तव्यमविरोधि यदौषधम्।। (सु.क.८/७५–७६)

Bite of Loota is very dreadful and very difficult to treat when there is less understanding of Loota. Loota had grown from the drops of perspiration of Holy Sage Vasishtha fallen on the cut grass.

Image 11.2

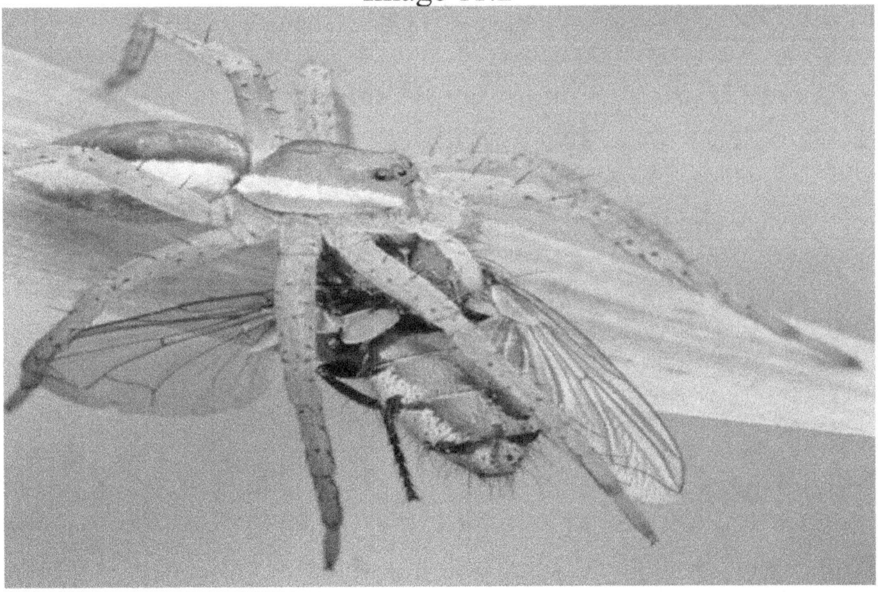

Table 11.19 Classification of Loota Visha

| Based on prognosis | -Kruchha Sadhya Loota: 8<br>- Asadhya Loota: 8 |
|---|---|
| Based on Doshaprakopa | -Vatika, Paittika, Shelshmika, Sannipatika. |
| Based on Visha Prabhava | -Mild: death occurs in 15 days.<br>- Moderate: death occurs in 10 days.<br>- Severe: death occurs in 7 days. |
| Based on site | • Swasa: Causes swelling with Jwara, burning sensation.<br>• Damshtra: Hard, firm, discolored site. Has swelling, pricking pain and burning sensation.<br>• Shakruta: Itching with pricking pain, burning sensation and foul smell.<br>• Mutra: Swelling with red edges, spreads outwards with burning sensation and foul smell.<br>• Shukra: Has hardness with burning sensation.<br>• Lalasrava: Elevated rash, mild pain, itching, soft to touch.<br>• Nakha: Burning sensation, itching and swelling feels as if hot smoke coming out.<br>• Artava: Has red swelling resembling garlands. |

- **Loota Damsha Samanya Lakshana:**

लूतादंशश्च सर्वोऽपि दद्रुमण्डलसन्निभः।।
सितोऽसितोऽरुणः पीतः श्यावो वा मृदुरुन्नतः।
मध्ये कृष्णोऽथवा श्यावः पर्यन्ते जालकावृतः।।
विसर्पवांस्छोफयुतस्तप्यते बहुवेदनः।
ज्वराशुपाकविक्लेदकोथावदरणान्वितः।।
क्लेदेन यत्स्पृशत्यङ्गं तत्रापि कुरुते व्रणम्।
(अ.हृ.उ.३७/५५–५८)

Mild rashes white, black, yellow or red in colour. Soft and raised up swelling with net like edges. Has burning sensation, severe pain, fever. Has quick suppuration with exudation.

Table 11.20 Day-vise signs and symptoms of Loota Visha

| | |
|---|---|
| Day 1: | सूचीव्यधवदाभाति ततोऽसौ प्रथमेऽहनि।<br>अव्यक्तवर्णः प्रचलः किञ्चित्कण्डूरुजान्वितः। (अ.स.उ.४४/१५)<br>• Pricking pain like needles<br>• No colour manifests, slightly painful.<br>• Itching and pain |
| Day 2: | द्वितीये त्युन्नतोऽन्तेषु पिटकैरिवचाचितः।<br>व्यक्तवर्णो नतो मध्ये कण्डूमान् ग्रन्थिसन्निभिः। (अ.स.उ.४४/१५)<br>• Edges are red surrounded by eruptions, depressed in the centre, itching, resembles a tumour. |
| Day 3: | तृतीये सज्वरो रोमहर्षकृद्रक्तमण्डलः।<br>शरावरूपस्तोदाढ्यो रोमकूपेषु सास्रवः। (अ.स.उ.४४/१५)<br>• Fever, horripilations, red patches in shape of Mandala. Severe pricking pain, bleeding from hair follicles. |
| Day 4: | महांश्चतुर्थे श्वयथुस्तापश्वासभ्रमप्रदः। (अ.स.उ.४४/१५)<br>• Profound swelling, temperature is raised.<br>• Dyspnoea, giddiness. |
| Day 5: | विकारान् कुरुते तांस्तान् पञ्चमे विषकोपजान। (अ.स.उ.४४/१५)<br>• Symptoms of poisoning related to the Dosha. |
| Day 6: | षष्ठे व्याप्नोति मर्माणि। (अ.स.उ.४४/१५)<br>• The poison invades all the vital organs. |
| Day 7: | सप्तमे हन्ति जीवितम्। (अ.स.उ.४४/१५)<br>• Whole body is affected and causes destruction of life. |

- **Loota Visha Chikitsa:**

Table 11.21

| | | |
|---|---|---|
| Dahana | अथाशु लूतादष्टस्यशस्त्रेण ादंशमुद्धरेत्द्य दहेत् जाम्बवोष्ठाद्यैर्न तु पित्तोतरं दहेत ।। (अ. स.उ.४४/२१) | Remove the sting from the site and cauterize with Jambavoshtha. |
| Lepa and Seka | लेपयेद्दग्धमगदैर्मधुसैन्धवसंयुतैःद्य सुशीतैः सेचयेत्र्यानु कषायैः क्षीरिवृक्षजैः।। (अ.स.उ.४४/२३) | The cauterized area be applied with Vishaghna Dravya with Madhu and Saindhava. Followed by Seka with Panchavalkala Kwatha. |

| Raktamokshana | सर्वतोऽपहरेद्रक्तं शृङ्गाद्यैः सिरयापि वा।<br>स्रुते रक्ते परीषेको घृतक्षिरादिभिर्हितः।। (अ.स.उ.४४/२४) | Done using Shrunga, Siravyadhana. Later pour cold ghee or cold milk. |
|---|---|---|
| Madhukadi Pana | मधूकं मधुकं कुष्ठं शिरीषोदीच्यपाटलाः।<br>सनिम्बसारिवाक्षौद्राः पानं लूताविषापहम।। (च.चि.२३/२०२) | • Ingredients: Madhooka, Madhuka, Kushtha, Shirisha, Udichya, Patala, Nimba, Sariva, Kshaudra.<br>• Indicated to drink for destruction of spider poison |

- **Spiders:**
  - Spider bites which harm humans are rare. Spiders bite only when they feel harmed or threatened. Their prey are usually small insects as their fangs are too small to penetrate human skin.
  - There are 60 different spider species but the most dangerous include: Black widow, brown recluses, hobo spiders.
  - The non-poisonous spider bites include: wolf spider bite, camel spider bite, jumping spider bite, banana spider bite.

Table 11.22 Classification, signs and symptoms of Spider poison

| **Black widow spider** | **Brown recluses spider** | **Hobo spiders** |
|---|---|---|
| Red hourglass shapes on their belly | Have a brown violin shaped mark on their head. | Have a grey V-shaped herringbone pattern on their bellies. |
| Difficulty in breathing, droopy eyes, swollen eyes. | Blister surrounded by reddish skin. Blister ruptures and forms scars. | Severe headache within minutes or hours of bite. |

| Headache, increased salivation, nausea, vomiting. | Itchy skin at the bite site.<br>Itchy skin all over the body. | Hardening of skin within 30 minutes of bite. |
|---|---|---|
| Profuse sweating, itchy skin rashes. | | Blisters with pus oozing. Red swollen skin. |
| Muscle cramps, stiffness of stomach, shoulders, chest, neck. | | Nausea, fatigue, memory problems. |

**Spider bite management:**

- Clean the bite area with soap and potable water.
- Apply damp wash cloth or ice pack at the site.
- Elevate the bitten area. Take antihistamine to ease itching and swelling.
- Anti venom  be given.
- Muscle relaxants, pain killers, sedatives.
- Daily cleaning with povidine-iodine solution to avoid second infections.
- Soaking the bitten area in Normal Saline 3 times a day.
- Seek immediate medical attention in case of severe symptoms

**3. Vrushchika Visha:**

Image 11.3

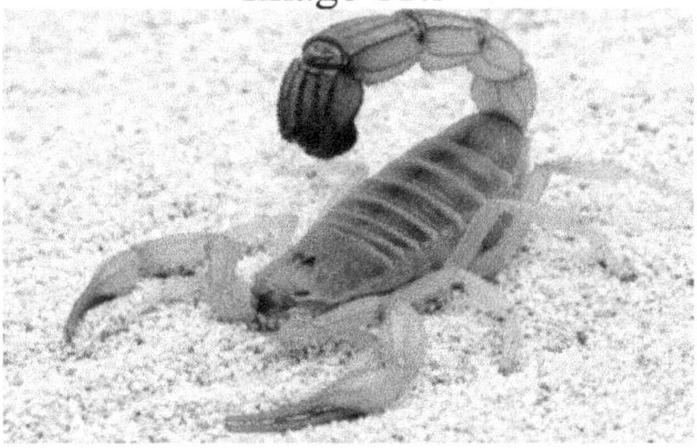

Table 11.23 Classification of Vrushchika

| Charak Samhita Chikitsa Sthana | 1. Dooshivishaja Vrushchika<br>2. Prana haram/ Asadhya |
|---|---|
| Sushruta Samhita Kalpa Sthana | 1. Mahavisha : 15 types<br>2. Madhyavisha: 3 types<br>3. Mandavisha: 12 types |
| Ashtanga Hridaya Uttartantra | 1. Mahavisha: strong poison<br>2. Madhyavisha: moderate poison<br>3. Mandavisha: mild poison |

Table 11.24 Features of Vrushchika by Acharya Sushruta

| **Mahavisha** | **Madhyavisha** | **Mandavisha** |
|---|---|---|
| White, brown, red body. | Red, yellow or brown body colour. | Body has the colour of cow's urine and is coarse. |
| Belly being either white, red, blue or yellow. | Belly is smoky in colour. | Belly has colour of red algae. |
| Has 2 joints in the tail. | Has 3 joints in the tail. | Has highest number of joints in the tail. |

- **Vrushchika Visha Samanya Lakshana:**

दहत्यग्निरिवादौ तु भिनत्तीवोर्ध्वमाशु च।
वृश्चिकस्य विषं याति दंशे पश्चात्तु तिष्ठति।। (च.चि.२३/१५०)

Initially the site of bite has severe burning sensation. The poison moves in upward direction very quickly and later gets stationary at the bite area.

Table 11.25 Symptoms produced by various Vrushchika

| Mahavisha | Vesicles, dizziness, burning sensation, fever, black blood flows out from the site of bite. |
|---|---|
| Madhyavisha | Fainting, swollen tongue, difficulty in swallowing. |
| Mandavisha | Pain, shivering, stiffness of body, black blood oozes from the bite area. |

Table 11.26 Damsha features according to Dosha

| | |
|---|---|
| Vataja Damsha | • Obstruction to upward movement of Vata causes pain in chest area. Dilated veins.<br>• Pain and swelling in joints.<br>• Body has blue discoloration and severe pain in calf muscles. |
| Pittaja Damsha | • Becomes unconsciousness, warm air expiration, burning sensation in heart region.<br>• Bitter taste in mouth, reddish-yellow swelling develops. |
| Kaphaja Damsha | • Nausea, vomiting, loss of appetite, excessive salivation.<br>• Sweet taste in mouth, runny nose, feeling cold. |

- **Asadhya Vrushchika Damsha Lakshana:**

  दष्टोऽसाध्यस्तु दृग्घ्राणरसनोपहतो नरः।
  मांसैः पतद्भिरत्यर्थं वेदनार्तो जहात्यसून।। (च.चि.२३/१५१)

Loss of vision, taste, smell, excessive flesh falling from bite area, excessive pain are symptoms of incurable Vrushchika Visha.

- **Vrushchika Visha Chikitsa:**

Table 11.27

| | |
|---|---|
| Tikshna Visha Vrushchika | • Pratisarana: with powders of Haridra, Saindhava, flowers of Shirisha.<br>• Lepa: Surasa, Gomutra, Matulunga juice.<br>• Pana: Ghrita with honey. |
| Madhyam Visha Vrushchika | • Pratisarana: Powders of Trikatu, Saindhava, flowers of Shirisha.<br>• Lepa: Surasa, Gomutra, juice of Matulunga.<br>• Pana: Milk with plenty of sugar. |
| Manda Visha Vrushchika | • Sechana: Chakra taila.<br>• Swedana: using anti-poisonous drugs.<br>• Pana: Cooled milk with jaggery. |

**Scorpion:**

- Scorpion is from class Arachnidae belongs to Anthropode. Scorpions have a front pair of claws and a flexible tail.
- The joint of tail has a communication with poisonous gland

which on stinging secrets venom.

- Most scorpion stings are harmless.
- < 5% requires medical attention.

Table 11.28 Systemic features of scorpion bite

| Grade 1 | Severe excruciating pain at the site of bite which radiates to corresponding dermatomes. |
|---|---|
| Grade 2 | Profuse sweating, salivation, hypotension or hypertension, cold extremities. |
| Grade 3 | Pulmonary oedema with hypotension or hypertension, cold extremities. |
| Grade 4 | Warm extremities, hypotension, tachycardia, pulmonary oedema, shock. |
| Grade 5 | Death occurs. |

**Scorpion bite management:**

- Apply tourniquet above the sting site.
- Incision and suction be done. Wash the site with weak solution of ammonia.
- Apply ice cold pack.
- Inject local anaesthetic to decrease the pain.
- IV fluids and oxygen as per the need.
- Specific anti venoms are available for most of the species.

**4. Mooshika Visha**

The Visha Adhishthan is Shukra.

Table 11.29 Types of Mooshika

| लालन | चपाल | पुत्रक |
|---|---|---|
| हसिर | चिकिर | अजिन |
| कषायदंत | कुलक | कोकिल |
| कपिल | असित | अरुण |

| शबल | श्वेत | कपोताभा |
|---|---|---|
| पलितउन्दुर | छुछुनदर | रसाला |

- Mooshika Visha Samanya Lakshana:

  आदंशाच्छोणितं पाण्डु मण्डलानि ज्वरोऽरुचिः।
  लोमहर्षश्च दाहश्चाप्याखुदूषीविषार्दित।। (च.चि.२३/१४७)

Pale blood coming out from the site of bite, rashes, fever, anorexia, horripilation, burning sensation.

भवन्ति चौषां दंशेषु ग्रन्थिमण्डलकर्णिकाः।
पिडकोपचयश्चोग्रः शोफश्च भृशदारुणः।। (सु.क.७/२७)

Tumours develop. Patches of small eruptions which are discolored, severe swelling.

- Mooshika Visha Asadhya Lakshana:

  मूर्च्छाङ्गशोथवैवर्ण्यक्लेदशब्दाश्रुतिज्वराः।
  शिरोगुरुत्वं लालासृक्छर्दिश्चासाध्यमूषिकैः।। (च.चि.२३/१४८)

Fainting, swelling of body parts, discoloration, moisture, deafness, fever, heaviness of head, salivation, hematemesis.

- Mooshika Visha Chikitsa:

  रसाञ्जनहरिद्रेन्द्रयवकट्वीषु वा कृतम्।
  प्रातः सातिविषं कल्कं लिह्यान्माक्षिकसंयुतम।।३९।।
  तण्डुलीयकमूलेषु सर्पिः सिद्धं पिबेन्नरः।
  आस्फोतमूलसिद्धं वा पञ्चकापित्थमेव वा।।
  (सु.क.७/३९–४०)

Juice of cow dung and Kapittha be added with honey be intaken. Powder of Rasanjana, Indrayava, Haridra, Katvi mixed with honey. Paste of Ativisha mixed with honey. Ghee boiled with Tanduliyaka, root of Asphota.

**General treatment of Mooshika Visha:**

- Cauterization at the bite site followed by blood letting.
- Later apply the paste of Shirisha, Haridra, Kushtha, Kesar.
- Vamana: macerate Shirisha, Madana, Devadali with curd to induce Vamana.
- Virechana: Triphala, Trivrutta, Danti paste.
- Nasya be done with fruits of Shirisha.
- Anjana: cow dung mixed with Trikatu.

**Rat bite:**

- Rat-bite fever (RBF) is a rare bacterial disease that spreads through the bite of infected rats. RBF can also spread if an infected rat scratches or when one come in contact with rat saliva, faeces, or urine.
- Caused by Streptobacillus moniliformis, Spirillum minus.

Table 11.30 Symptoms of rat bite fever

| | |
|---|---|
| Streptobacillus moniliformis | • Headache, nausea, vomiting, fever, skin rashes around hands and feet.<br>• Joint pain, muscle pain.<br>• Symptoms occur after 3-10 days of exposure. |
| Spirillum minus | • Recurrent fever, skin lesions around bite, swollen lymph nodes, rashes on whole body. |

- Complications: Meningitis, myocarditis, endocarditis, pericarditis, nephritis, hepatitis, pneumonia.

**Rat bite fever management:**

- Wash the wound with soap and potable water. Pat dry with a damp towel.

- Antibiotics: penicillin, ceftriaxone, ampicillin, amoxicillin or doxycycline.
- For allergies: erythromycin, tetracycline be used.

## 5. Alarka Visha

***Nidana and Samprapti:***

श्वशृगालतरक्ष्वृक्षव्याघ्रादीनां यदाऽनिलः।
श्लेष्मप्रदुष्टो मुष्णाति सञ्ज्ञां सञ्ज्ञावहाश्रितः।।
तदा प्रस्रस्तलाङ्गूलहनुस्कन्धोऽतिलालवान्।
अत्यर्थबधिरोऽन्धश्च सोऽन्योन्यमभिधावति।।
तेनोन्मत्तेन दष्टस्य दंष्ट्रिणा सविषेण त।
सुप्तता जायते दंशे कृष्णं चातिस्रवत्यसृक।।
दिग्धविद्धस्य लिङ्गेन प्रायशश्चोपलक्षितः। (सु.क.७/४३–४६)

- When Vata and Kapha gets aggravated in the body of dog, fox, jackal like animals it get accumulated in the sense organs.
- The animal has loss of sensation. Runs around very much, tail is curled between two legs, lower jaw dropped and excessive salivation, gets deaf and blind.
- When such an animal bites human, there occurs loss of sensation, black discoloration and heavy bleeding at the site of bite.
- The person if observes image of animal in water or mirror, it may be considered as fatal.

**Shva Damsha Lakshana:**

श्वा त्रिदोषप्रकोपात्तु तथा धातुविपर्ययात्।
शिरोऽभितापी लालास्राव्यधोवक्त्रस्तथा भवेत्।। (च.चि.२३/१७५)

Vitiation of Tridosha, headache, salivation, dropped face.

**Shva Damsha Asadhya Lakshana:**

येन चापि भवेद्दष्टस्तस्य चेष्टां रुतं नरः।।
बहुशः प्रतिकुर्वाणः क्रियाहीनो विनश्यति।
दंष्ट्रिणा येन दष्टश्च तद्रूपं यस्तु पश्यति।।
अप्सु वा यदि वाऽऽदर्शेऽरिष्टं तस्य विनिर्दिशेत्।
(सु.क.७/४६.४८)

- Person if observes the animal image in water, mirror shows fatality.
- If person becomes afraid even by seeing or touching water known as hydrophobia. This shows fatal condition.

**Shva Damsha Chikitsa:**

दंशं विस्राव्य तैर्दष्टे सर्पिषा परिदाहितम्।।
प्रदिह्यादगदैः, सर्पिः पुराणं पाययेत च।
अर्कक्षीरयुतं ह्यस्य दद्याच्चापि विशोधनम।।
श्वेतां पुनर्नवां चास्य दद्याद्धत्तूरकायुताम्।
पललं तिलतैलं च रूपिकायाः पयो गुडः।।
निहन्ति विषमालर्क मेघवृन्दमिवानिलः।
मूलस्य शरपुङ्खायाः कर्षं धत्तूरकार्धिकम्।।
तण्डुलोदकमादाय पेषयेत्तण्डुलैः सह।
उन्मत्तकस्य पत्रैस्तु संवेष्ट्यापूपकं पचेत्।।
खादेदौषधकाले तमलर्कविषदूषितः।
करोति श्वविकारांस्तु तस्मिञ्जीर्यति चौषध।।
विकाराः शिशिरे याप्या गृहे वारिविवर्जित।
ततः शान्तविकारस्तु स्नात्वा चौवापरेऽहनि।।
शालिषष्टिकयोर्भक्तं क्षीरेणोष्णेन भोजयेत्।
दिनत्रये पञ्चमे वा विधिरेषोऽर्धमात्रया।।
कर्तव्यो भिषजाऽवश्यमलर्कविषनाशनः।
कुप्येत् स्वयं विषं यस्य न स जीवति मानवः।।
तस्मात् प्रकोपयेदाशु स्वयं यावत् प्रकुप्यति। (सु.क.७/५१–५६)

- Blood containing poison should be sucked from the site of bite. Later hot ghee should be poured on the site.
- Anti poisonous medicines be made into poultice and applied at bite area.
- Purana Ghrita be drank. Tila taila mixed with sap of Arka be given for purgation.
- Sap of Arka with jaggery when consumed cures rabid dog poison.
- Root of Sharpunkh:10gm, Dhattura root:5gm, Tandula and Tandulodaka be macerated. Cover this ball with leaves of Dhattura and make Apupa. Consume this during meal time.
- If after consuming this Apupa, person performs animal activities, he should be confined in a cold room with no water.
- When the person becomes normal, should take bath next day. Consume meals having rice and milk for 3-5 days.

**Rabies:**

- Rabies virus (RABV) is transmitted through direct contact with saliva or brain or nervous system tissue from an infected animal. Rabies is fatal but preventable. It can spread to people and pets if they are bitten or scratched by a rabid animal.
- People undergo 4 phases: Incubation, prodromal phase, acute neurologic phase, coma.

Table 11.31 Symptoms of rabies virus

| | |
|---|---|
| Prodromal phase | • Fever, tiredness, cough, sore throat, muscle pain.<br>• Nausea, vomiting, diarrhoea.<br>• Burning sensation, numbness, tingling, itching around the site of bite. |
| Acute neurologic furious phase | • Agitation and aggression, seizures, hallucination, muscle twitching.<br>• Fever, tachycardia, hyperventilation, excessive salivation.<br>• Anisocoria (different pupil sizes), facial palsy, delirium.<br>• Hydrophobia, aerophobia. |

| Acute neurologic paralytic phase | • Fever, headache, neck stiffness.<br>• Weakness of body part bitten which progresses to other body parts.<br>• Tingling sensation, paralysis, coma. |
|---|---|

- **Diagnosis:** Skin biopsy, saliva test, CSF test, blood test, MRI.

- **Treatment:**
  - Clean the wound gently yet thoroughly with soap and potable water.
  - Rabies vaccine: 1st vaccine as soon ass possible after exposure. Additional doses on days 3, 7, 14 after the first. If previously immunized person bitten than, 2 doses given 1 week apart. If previous exposure is beyond 3 years, complete immunization schedule should be followed.
  - Human Rabies Immune Globulin (HRIG): Given near the wound to destroy virus upto the time immune system takes over.

**6. Keeta Visha:**

- ***Origin of insects:***

सर्पाणामेव विण्मूत्रशुक्राण्डशवकोथजाः।
दोषैर्व्यस्तैः समस्तैश्च युक्ताः कीटाश्चतुर्विधाः।। (अ.हृ.उ.३७/१)

Insects are born from faeces, urine, semen, eggs or carcass of snakes.

- **Keeta Bheda:** Vataja, Pittaja, Kaphaja, Sannipataja.

- **Keeta Damsha Samanya Lakshana:**

वेगाश्च सर्पवच्छोफो वर्धिष्णुर्विस्त्ररक्तता।।
शिरोक्षिगौरवं मूर्च्छा भ्रमः श्वासोऽतिवेदना।
सर्वेषां कर्णिका शोफो ज्वरः कण्डूररोचकः।। (अ.हृ.उ.३७/४–५)

Swelling increases in size, foul smell from blood, heaviness of head and eyes, fainting, giddiness, dyspnoea, sever pain at the site of bite, fever, itching, loss of appetite.

Table 11.32 Dosha wise symptoms of Keeta Visha

| **Vataja** | **Pittaja** | **Kaphaja** | **Sannipataja** |
|---|---|---|---|
| Pricking pain, increased pain intensity at the site of bite. | Slight exudation, severe burning sensation, redness, swelling resembles the fruit of Peelu. | Mild pain, swelling resembles the fruit of Udumbara. | Has copious amount of exudation. |

- Visha Yukta Keeta Damsha Lakshana:

कण्डूनिस्तोदवैवर्ण्यसुप्तिक्लेदोपशोषणम्।
विदाहरागरुक्पाकाः शोफो ग्रन्थिनिकुञ्चनम।।
दंशावदरणं स्फोटाः कर्णिका मण्डलानि च।
ज्वरश्च सविषे लिङ्गं विपरीतं तु निर्विष।।
(च.चि.२३/१७७–१७८)

Itching, piercing pain, discoloration, numbness, moisture increased, drying heat, oedema associated with burning sensation, redness, pain, suppuration, swelling, cyst formation, flesh tearing down, boils, rashes, fever.

- **Keeta Visha Chikitsa:**

Table 11.33 Treatment measures for Keeta Visha

| Lepa | क्षीरिवृक्षत्वगालेपः शुद्धे कीटविषापहः।। (च.चि.२३/१९९) मुक्तालेपो वरः शोथदाहतोदज्वरापहः। (च.चि. २३/२००) | Kshiri Vruksha Twag (bark) Lepa be applied. Muktika is good for decreasing swelling, burning sensation, pricking pain, fever. |
|---|---|---|

| | | |
|---|---|---|
| Agadapana | वचा हिङ्गु विडङ्गानि सैन्धवं गजपिप्पली।।२७।।<br>पाठा प्रतिविषा व्योषं काश्यपेन विनिर्मितम्।<br>दशाङ्गमगदं पीत्वा सर्वकीटविषं जयेत्।। (अ.हृ.उ.३७/२७–२८) | Vacha, Hingu, Vidanga, Saindhava, Gajapippali, Patha, Prativisha, Vyosha be made into pills and used. Cures all types of insect poisons. |

## 7. Vector borne diseases:

Vector-borne diseases are caused by the bites of disease-causing pathogens like mosquitoes and ticks. These organisms first get infected by the disease-causing pathogens, and once infected, they can transmit the pathogen to humans throughout their life whenever they come in contact with a human host.

Table 11.34

| Diseases | Cause | Symptoms |
|---|---|---|
| Chikungunya | Virus carried by Aedes mosquito | Sudden fever, joint pain, muscle aches, headache, nausea, fatigue, skin rashes. |
| Yellow fever | Virus carried by Aedes mosquito | Fever, muscle pain, chills, headache, nausea.<br>Fatal symptoms: gastric bleeding, jaundice, dark urine, abdominal pain. |
| Dengue | Virus carried by Aedes mosquito | Sudden high fever, severe headache, retro-orbital pain, joint pain, muscle pain, nausea, vomiting, swollen lymph nodes. |
| Malaria | Parasite caused by Anopheles mosquito | Fever, chills, sweating, headache, bodyache, nausea, vomiting, diarrhoea, breathing abnormality. |
| Japanese encephalitis | Virus transmitted by Culex mosquito | Fever, headache vomiting, neurological symptoms, weakness, movement issues after some days. Seizures in children. |
| Chagas disease | Parasite transmitted by Triatomine bugs | Fever, headache, bodyache, fatigue, nausea, enlarged lymph nodes, skin rashes. |

| Sleeping sickness | Parasite carried by Tsetse flies | Fever, chills, headache, muscle pain, joint pain, skin rash, anaemia, swollen lymph nodes, drowsiness, unable to concentrate, difficulty in walking and speech. |
|---|---|---|
| Plague | Bacteria transmitted from rats to humans by fleas | -Bubonic plague: swollen lymph nodes, filling sores with pus.<br>-Pneumonic plague: shortness of breath, chest pain, cough, bloody sputum. |

***Treatment:***

- Vaccines be taken for yellow fever, Japanese encephalitis, tick-borne encephalitis.
- There's no stagnant water around the residence as it is the breeding ground for vectors.
- Apply insect repellents and cover as much as possible to avoid bites of insects.
- Avoid touching infected people and animal's blood or fluids.

**Multiple Choice Questions**

**1. Acharya Sushruta mentions how many numbers of Mandali Sarpa ?**

A. 20 B. 22 C. 12 D. 16

**2. How many Sarpa Visha Vega are mentioned?**

A. 5 B. 8 C. 7 D. 9

**3. Which of the following is a musculotoxic snake?**

A. Sea snake B. Pit viper C. Krait D. Coral cobra

**4. Red patches in the shape of Mandala: occurs on which day of Loota Visha?**

A. 2nd B. 4th C. 3rd D. 1st

**5. Chagas disease is transmitted by ?**

A. Triatomine bugs B. Tsetse flies C. Aedes mosquito D. Culex

**6.** मूर्च्छाङ्गशोथवैवर्ण्यक्लेदशब्दाश्रुतिज्वराः। **is which Visha Asadhya Lakshana?**

A. Sarpa Visha　　B. Keeta Visha
C. Mooshika Visha　　D. Alarka Visha

**7. Which Vrushchika has 3 joints in the tail?**

A. Mahavisha　　B. Madhyavisha
C. Mandavisha　　D. All types

**8. PAV each vial has what amount of neutralized snake venom?**

A. 1-5mg　B. 20-24mg　C. 6-8mg　D. 10-12mg

**9. Pittaja Keeta Visha resembles which fruit?**

A. Udumbara　B. Peelu　C. Nimba　D. Jambu

**10. What is the fatal dose of King cobra venom?**

A. 5-8mg　B. 12-15mg　C. 1-3mg　D. 7-9mg

**11. Darvikara Sarpa aggravates which Dosha?**

A. Tridosha　B. Kapha　C. Vata　D. Pitta

**12. Venom of which poisonous snake is not used in hyper-immunizing a horse to prepare PAV?**

A. Common krait　　B. Russell's viper
C. Sea snake　　D. Saw scaled viper

**13. Bindu Lekha Vichitranga is identification feature for which snake?**

A. Darvikara　B. Mandali　C. Rajimana　D. Nirvisha

**14.** मुक्तालेपो वरः शोथदाहतोदज्वरापहः| **is Chikitsa for which Jangama Visha?**

A. Sarpa　B. Keeta　C. Loota　D. Vrushchika

**15. Loss of vision due to mydriasis is a symptom of which snake poisoning?**

A. Cobra
B. King cobra
C. Russell's viper
D. Pit viper

**Answer key for MCQs:**

| | |
|---|---|
| 1 | B |
| 2 | C |
| 3 | A |
| 4 | C |
| 5 | A |
| 6 | C |
| 7 | B |
| 8 | C |

| | |
|---|---|
| 9 | B |
| 10 | B |
| 11 | C |
| 12 | C |
| 13 | C |
| 14 | B |
| 15 | A |

# Ch. 12
# Kritrima Visha

## 12.1 Inorganic Acids:

### *1. Sulphuric Acid:*

- Also known as oil of vitriol. Has compounds Hydrogen, Sulphur, Oxygen.
- It is heavy, oily, colourless, odourless, non fuming liquid and hygroscopic.

- **Fatal dose:** 5-10 ml
- **Fatal period:** 12-18 hours

Table 12.1

| | |
|---|---|
| **Signs and symptoms** | • Severe pain on contact and severe burns occur.<br>• Tissue damage occurs, hematemesis, skin drainage and pain.<br>• Eye burning, eye pain, vision loss.<br>• Chest pain, difficulty in breathing, shortness of breath.<br>• Bluish skin, nails, lips.<br>• Tachycardia, rapid fall of blood pressure. |
| **Treatment** | • Wash with water immediately if contact with skin or eyes.<br>• Apply thick paste of magnesium oxide.<br>• Dress the wounds, antibiotics be taken to avoid secondary infection. |
| **Post-mortem appearance** | • Corrosion of oral cavity, tongue, throat, chin and possibly hand.<br>• Chalky white teeth.<br>• Stomach perforation in severe cases.<br>• Corroded area appears brown or black. |

| Medico-legal aspects | • Vitriolage is commonly done by corrosive acids.<br>• Accidental poisoning in children or laboratory.<br>• Rarely homicidal or suicidal poisoning.<br>• Used to procure abortion. |
|---|---|

- Vitriolage: Intentional act of throwing corrosives on face or body with a intention to disfigure. Commonly done by oil of vitriol. So it is called as Vitriolage.

*2. Hydrochloric Acid:*

- Also known as Spirit of Salts, Muriatic acid.
- Colourless, odourless, volatile, fuming liquid.
- May acquire yellowish tinge on exposing to air.

- **Fatal dose:** 15-18 ml
- **Fatal period:** 18-30 hours

Table 12.2

| Signs and symptoms | • Does not stain but in strong doses causes corrosion.<br>• Fume inhalation causes respiratory irritation.<br>• Doesn't cause perforation.<br>• Shock occurs. |
|---|---|
| **Treatment** | • ABC maintenance.<br>• Remove the clothing from affected area and wash with plenty of water.<br>• Don't induce emesis. Intake 4-8 ounces of milk or water.<br>• Maintain respiratory and cardiovascular functions. |
| **Post-mortem appearance** | • Skin and mucous membrane shows corrosion. Skin becomes brownish coloured and parchment paper like.<br>• Coagulation in mucous membrane of: tongue, pharynx, oesophagus.<br>• Stomach becomes soft, oedematous, congestion and has ulcers.<br>• Stomach contents has blood mixed with mucous.<br>• Inflammation and oedema of respiratory tract. |

*2. Nitric Acid:*

- Also known as Aqua fortis, Red spirit of Nitre.
- It is a clear, colourless, fuming liquid with pungent smell.
- Gives yellowish discoloration.

- **Fatal dose:** 10-15 ml
- **Fatal period:** 12-24 hours

Table 12.3

| | |
|---|---|
| **Signs and symptoms** | • Lips, tongue and mucous membrane become white and soft. Later become yellowish.<br>• Yellowish teeth discoloration.<br>• Abdominal pain, distention, tenderness.<br>• Irritation to eyes, congestion of throat on fumes inhalation. |
| **Treatment** | • ABC support.<br>• For fume inhalation: expose to fresh air and give oxygen support.<br>• Give 4 ounces of milk of magnesia. |
| **Post-mortem appearance** | • Corrosion of skin, angle of mouth, mucous membrane with yellowish discoloration.<br>• Stomach wall becomes soft and friable.<br>• Perforation is less common. |

## 12.2 Organic Acids:

*4. Oxalic Acid:*

- It was first isolated from the flowering plant of genus Oxalis.
- An organic acid named ethanedioic acid. It is the simplest dicarboxylic acid.
- It is a white crystal solid which forms a colourless solution with water.
- It is a colourless, odourless, transparent, prismatic crystals resembling crystals of magnesium sulphate.
- Also known as Salts of Sorrel, Acid of sugar.
- It has a sour slightly bitter acidic taste.

- **Fatal dose:** 15-20 grams

- **Fatal period:** 1-2 hours

Table 12.4

| | |
|---|---|
| **Signs and symptoms** | • Local: Corrosion of mucosa which appears scalded.<br>• Systemic: Vomiting, diarrhoea, hypocalcaemia, tenderness, cramps, convulsions, metabolic acidosis, renal failure, uraemia.<br>• Chvostek's sign: By tapping on facial nerve, it causes spasm of facial muscles. |
| **Treatment** | • Local: Wash the affected area with plenty of water.<br>• Systemic: Gastric lavage with calcium gluconate.<br>• IV calcium gluconate.<br>• Symptomatic treatment. |
| **Post-mortem appearance** | • Scalded mucosa of GIT.<br>• Scalded bleachy appearance of mouth, tongue, pharynx, oesophagus.<br>• Renal tubules congestion with oxalate crystals present. |
| **Medico-legal aspects** | • Accidental poisoning: common.<br>• Homicidal poisoning and suicidal poisoning. |
| **Uses** | • Bleaching agent, cleaning agent for brass and copper articles. |

***5. Carbolic Acid:***

- Also known as Phenol, Benzenol, Phenolic acid.
- It is a white crystalline solid which is volatile.
- Colourless, prismatic and needle like crystals.
- Crystals turn pink and liquefies when exposed to air.
- Concentrated phenol has a dark brown colour with cresol like impurities.
- Lysol is 50% solution of cresol. Dettol is chlorinated phenol with terpineol. Phenyl consists of 5% phenol in water.

- **Fatal dose:** 25-50 ml
- **Fatal period:** 3-4 hours

Table 12.5

| | |
|---|---|
| **Signs and symptoms** | • Local: Has burning pain, tingling sensation, numbness, anaesthesia.<br>• Produces white stain which falls within some days leaving brown stain.<br>• Systemic: Nausea, vomiting, hepatic failure.<br>• Slow and forceful respiration.<br>• Headache, giddiness, convulsions, unconsciousness, coma.<br>• Urine is colourless but becomes green on contact with air as oxidation of phenol metabolites. |
| **Treatment** | • Skin: wash with un-diluted polyethylene glycol.<br>• Give oxygen therapy.<br>• Stomach wash with magnesium sulphate with precaution.<br>• Lidocaine for ventricular arrhythmia, benzodiazepines to treat convulsions. |
| **Post-mortem appearance** | • Corrosion at lips, angle of mouth, chin. Has white scars initially later turns brown.<br>• Splashing may be observed. Phenol smell may be found.<br>• Tongue becomes white and swollen. Mucosa of GIT becomes hard and greyish white with longitudinal folds and leathery appearance.<br>• Urine on exposure to air turns green coloured. |
| **Medico-legal aspects** | • Accidental poisoning, suicidal poisoning or homicidal poisoning. |
| **Uses** | • As an antiseptic, disinfectant.<br>• To make plastics, resin, epoxy. |

### *6. Formic Acid:*

- Also known as Formylic acid and Methanoic acid.
- Commonly used in leather manufacturing and so easily available in market.
- It is a colourless, pungent liquid. It is severely known to burn skin.

- **Fatal dose:** 50-200 ml
- **Fatal period:** 12-15 hours

Table 12.6

| | |
|---|---|
| **Signs and symptoms** | • Retrosternal burning, abdominal pain, chest pain.<br>• Headache, dizziness, nausea, vomiting, dysphagia, oesophageal strictures.<br>• On eye exposure, causes severe irritation and burns. Possibly eye damage.<br>• Hematuria, hematemesis, septicaemia, hypotension.<br>• Gastrointestinal perforation, respiratory problems. |
| **Treatment** | • Emesis should be avoided.<br>• Demulcents be used.<br>• IV Sodium bicarbonate during initial hours reduces fatality.<br>• Antidote: Fomepizole.<br>• Folinic acid: 1mg/kg IV 4 hourly for 6 doses.<br>• Dialysis. |
| **Uses** | • As a disinfectant and to make plastic. |

## 12.3 Alkalies

***7. Potassium hydroxide:***

- Also known as Caustic potash and Potassium hydrate.
- Odourless, white flaky substance soluble in water.

Table 12.7

| | |
|---|---|
| **Signs and symptoms** | • Highly corrosive and on contact with skin causes burning sensation.<br>• On eye contact causes irritation and eye damage.<br>• Headache, dizziness, nausea, vomiting.<br>• Inhalation can cause irritation of lungs and pulmonary oedema.<br>• Skin allergy, irritates nose and throat. |
| **Treatment** | • On eye contact: wash with plenty of water by lifting upper and lower eye lids for 30 minutes. Remove contact lenses while washing eyes.<br>• On skin contact: wash the area with plenty of water and remove the residual amount. Remove the contaminated clothes.<br>• ABC care.<br>• Fluid through IV in case of headache, vomiting, etc. |

| Uses | • Making alkaline batteries, electroplating.<br>• In paints and varnish removers. |
|---|---|

**8. Sodium hydroxide:**

- Also known as Caustic soda, Soda lye, Sodium hydrate.
- It is a white, non-combustible solid which absorbs moisture from the air.
- It is odourless making it more dangerous, as it doesn't give signals for harmful levels.

Table 12.8

| Signs and symptoms | • Highly irritating and corrosive. Causes permanent tissue damage on contact.<br>• Causes hydrolysis of protein causing severe burns in eyes.<br>• Inhalation causes laryngitis and pulmonary oedema.<br>• Drooling, stridor, abdominal pain, vomiting, perforation of GI tract. |
|---|---|
| Treatment | • Remove the contaminated clothing. Wash the site with plenty of water.<br>• IV fluid, respiratory and cardiovascular support be given. |
| Uses | • To make soaps, detergents, drain cleaner to unclog pipes, paper industry. |

## 12.4 Asphyxiants:

***9. Carbon monoxide:***

- It is a colourless, odourless, tasteless, non-irritant gas.
- Lighter than air, burns with blue flame, soluble in water.
- It is found from incomplete combustion of wood, charcoal, kerosene.
- Automobile exhaust, tobacco smoke, mines

Table 12.9

| | |
|---|---|
| **Signs and symptoms** | • Carbon monoxide reacts 200 times more with Hb than oxygen causing anaemic type of hypoxia.<br>• 0-10% No specific symptoms.<br>• 10-20% Exertional breathlessness, weakness, headache.<br>• 20-30% Severe headache, decreased memory, irritability, rapid fatigue.<br>• 30-40% Decreased vision, confusion, dizziness, nausea, vomiting.<br>• 40-50% Increased confusion, ataxia, rapid respiration. Symptoms resemble alcohol intoxication.<br>• 50-60% Coma with intermittent convulsions, tachycardia with weak pulse, reddish skin discoloration.<br>• 60-70% Increased depth of coma and incontinence of urine and faeces.<br>• 70-80% Absent reflexes, feeble pulse, shallow respiration, death occurs.<br>• >80% Immediate death from respiratory failure. |
| **Treatment** | • Remove the patient from affected environment.<br>• Hyperbaric oxygenation treatment.<br>• Benzodiazepines for convulsions, mannitol for cerebral oedema.<br>• Decreased activities to avoid risk of cerebral demyelination. |
| **Post-mortem appearance** | • Pinkish colour of skin, mucosa, pinkish post-mortem lividity.<br>• Blisters on dependent parts like buttocks, knee, wrists.<br>• Froth at nostrils and mouth, features of asphyxia, pulmonary oedema.<br>• Blood and internal organs are pinkish red.<br>• Petechial haemorrhage in white matter and putamen.<br>• Necrosis of globus pallidus. |
| **Medico-legal aspects** | • Accidental poisoning. |

### *10. Carbon dioxide:*

- Heavy, odourless, colourless gas. In solid form known as Dry ice.
- Its sources are combustion, mines, exhalation, manholes,

wells, cellar.

Table 12.10

| | |
|---|---|
| **Signs and symptoms** | • Headache, dizziness, confusion, nausea, vomiting.<br>• Dyspnoea, tachycardia, hypertension.<br>• Convulsions, paralysis of respiratory centre. |
| **Treatment** | • Remove the patient from areas of carbon dioxide sources.<br>• Give hyperbaric oxygenation therapy.<br>• Supportive treatments, cardiovascular support. |
| **Post-mortem appearance** | • Cyanosis, congestion, froth at nostrils and mouth.<br>• Petechial haemorrhage, venous engorgement, dark coloured blood. |
| **Medico-legal aspects** | • Accidental poisoning in workers working in deep wells, dampen pit, mines. |

## 12.5 Non-metallic poisons:

### *11. Phosphorous:*

- White, yellow, red phosphorus are available.

- **Fatal dose:** 60-120 mg
- **Fatal period:** 4-10 hours

- **Mechanism of action:**

Hepatotoxic, cardio toxic, causes fatty liver infiltration, necrosis of kidney. On skin contact causes irritation and burns the skin, mucosa.

- **Absorption, metabolism, excretion:**

Can be easily absorbed from stomach when there are fatty foods present. On absorption, it is retained in all organs and metabolized to hypo-phosphate. Excreted by urine, faeces, expired air.

Table 12.11

| | |
|---|---|
| **Signs and symptoms** | • Acute poisoning:<br>• Stage 1: Vomiting, diarrhoea, abdominal pain, garlic odour in vomitus, faeces is luminous in the dark.<br>• Stage 2: Symptoms subside.<br>• Stage 3: Symptoms reappear. Tender, enlarged liver, jaundice, hepatic failure, pruritus, encephalopathy, convulsions, renal failure.<br>• Chronic poisoning:<br>• Nausea, vomiting, diarrhoea, abdominal discomfort, eructation.<br>• Toothache, gingivitis, sloughing of gums, necrosis, sequestration, osteomyelitis of mandible (glass jaw).<br>• Anaemia, jaundice, wasting and weakness of muscles. |
| **Treatment** | • Avoid intake of fatty foods as it increases absorption of phosphorus.<br>• Gastric lavage with potassium permanganate (1:5000).<br>• Vitamin K, Calcium gluconate for hypoglycaemia.<br>• IV fluids, benzodiazepines for convulsions. |
| **Post-mortem appearance** | • Petechial haemorrhage, jaundice.<br>• Garlicky odour from gastric contents.<br>• Gastric mucosa turns greenish, yellowish and becomes soft.<br>• Gastric contents are luminous in the dark.<br>• Liver is enlarged, doughy, yellowish.<br>• Voluntary muscles show fatty degeneration.<br>• On microscopy, hepatocellular necrosis, cholestasis found. |
| **Medico-legal aspects** | • Accidental poisoning, suicidal poisoning, homicidal poisoning. |

## *12. Cyanide:*

Table 12.12

| | |
|---|---|
| **Signs and symptoms** | • Headache, dizziness, nausea, hypotension, dyspnoea, drowsiness, convulsions, cyanosis.<br>• Unconsciousness, froth at the mouth, respiratory failure.<br>• Specific bitter almond odour. |

| Treatment | • Start resuscitation immediately.<br>• Supportive measures be taken.<br>• Antidote: Amylnitrite + Sodium nitrite, Sodium thiosulphate. |
|---|---|

## 12.6 Hydrocarbons:

### *13. Kerosene:*

- These are substances which are exclusively made of hydrogen and carbon atoms.
- Substances made from hydrocarbons emit CO2, water, heat when combusted.

- **Fatal dose:** >10 ml
- **Fatal period:** Few hours

Table 12.13

| **Signs and symptoms** | • Burning sensation in mouth, pharynx.<br>• Nausea, vomiting, giddiness, blurry vision, cyanosis, dyspnoea.<br>• Drowsiness leading to stupor, coma, death.<br>• Mild tachypnoea, pulmonary oedema. |
|---|---|
| **Diagnosis** | • Chest X- ray for aspiration pneumonia. |
| **Treatment** | • Suction the secretions from airway.<br>• Evaluate and maintain oxygenation.<br>• Liquid paraffin + smashed banana: delays absorption.<br>• Avoid gastric lavage due to risk of aspiration.<br>• Antibiotics, corticosteroids. |
| **Post-mortem appearance** | • Acute gastroenteritis, signs of asphyxia.<br>• Typical kerosene odour from stomach contents.<br>• Degenerative changes in liver, kidney.<br>• Pulmonary oedema and bronchopneumonia found. |
| **Medico-legal aspects** | • Accidental poisoning in children.<br>• Suicidal poisoning occasionally.<br>• Homicidal poisoning in dowry cases. |

## 12.7 Agrochemical poisoning:

### *14. Organophosphorus compounds:*

- **Fatal dose:**
  Melathion: 60gm
  TEPP: 100gm
  OMPA: 175gm
  HETP: 300gm
- **Fatal period:** 24 hours

Table 12.14

| | |
|---|---|
| **Signs and symptoms** | • Nausea, vomiting, diarrhoea, abdominal pain.<br>• Increased bronchial secretions, lacrimation, sweating, cramps.<br>• Blurred vision, pin-point pupil, confusion, convulsions, coma. |
| **Treatment** | • Remove the contaminated cloths, wash with plenty of soap and water.<br>• Artificial respiration, resuscitation.<br>• Oxygenation should be maintained.<br>• Antidote: Atropine sulphate 2mg IV / 10 minutes upto atropinisation. |
| **Post-mortem appearance** | • Froth at mouth and nostrils, cyanosis, constricted pupil.<br>• Stomach contents has insecticide odour.<br>• Pulmonary oedema, cerebral oedema.<br>• Toxic myocarditis. |
| **Medico-legal aspects** | • Accidental poisoning, suicidal poisoning, homicidal poisoning. |

### *15. Carbamate poisoning;*

- Common insecticide substances. These increase muscarinic activities and show some nicotinic actions.

Table 12.15

| | |
|---|---|
| **Signs and symptoms** | • Acute: Salivation, sweating, urination, defecation, lacrimation, vomiting, miosis, bronchorrhea.<br>• Tachycardia, weakness, fasciculation, sweating, abdominal pain.<br>• Delayed: Proximal weakness, respiratory muscle weakness.<br>• Cured in 2-3 weeks. |
| **Treatment** | • Stabilization be done initially.<br>• For local contact use plenty of water to clean.<br>• On ingestion, activated charcoal be given within 1 hour.<br>• Gastric emptying done with intubation to avoid aspiration.<br>• 2-5mg IV Atropine to relieve bronchospasm and bronchorrhea. Dose can be doubled every 5 minutes if required. The dose is 0.05mg/kg in children.<br>• Diazepam to cure convulsions.<br>• Prophylactic diazepam to avoid neurocognitive problems after poisoning. |

### *16. Organo-chlorine compounds:*

- Insecticides, solvents, fumigants which are widely used contain OC compounds.
- Either cause CNS depression or stimulation depending on substance and dose.

- **Fatal dose:** 5-6 gm
- **Fatal period:** >1 hour

Table 12.16

| | |
|---|---|
| **Signs and symptoms** | • CNS depression and stimulation, euphoria, auditory and visual hallucination, convulsions, agitation, lethargy, unconsciousness.<br>• Nausea, vomiting, anorexia, confusion, tremor, myoclonus, respiratory depression.<br>• Unusual odour: turpentine, sulphur.<br>• Ear, nose, throat irritation, blurred vision, cough, acute lung ailments.<br>• Hepatotoxicity, renal toxicity, fatigue, twitching, dermatitis, headache. |
| **Laboratory investigation** | • RBS, Sr. Electrolyte, KFT, LFT, ABG analysis. |
| **Treatment** | • Supportive care for avoiding end organ damage.<br>• No specific antidote is available.<br>• On local contact, clean with soap and water. Remove the contaminated clothing.<br>• Multiple Dose Activated Charcoal. |
| **Post-mortem appearance** | • Insecticide like smell from stomach contents.<br>• Congestion of organs. |
| **Medico-legal aspects** | • Accidental poisoning, suicidal poisoning, homicidal poisoning. |

***17. Aluminium phosphide:***

- It is available in various fumigating substances and is highly toxic when inhaled from a freshly opened container.
- 
- **Fatal dose:** 0.15-05 gm
- **Fatal period:** 1 hour – 4 days

Table 12.17

| | |
|---|---|
| **Signs and symptoms** | • The signs and symptoms are non specific, dose dependent and increases with time.<br>• Direct effect on cardiomyocytes, fluid loss, renal gland damage.<br>• Dizziness, fatigue, chest tightness, headache, jaundice, nausea, vomiting, diarrhoea.<br>• Ataxia, numbness, paraesthesia, tremor, muscle weakness.<br>• Double vision (diplopia), Acute Respiratory Distress Syndrome (ARDS), arrhythmias, heartbeat abnormalities, coma. |
| **Treatment** | • Supportive therapy like resuscitation, oxygen therapy, maintenance of blood pressure.<br>• Use of $MgSO_4$. |

## *12.8 Household poisons:*

- When poisoning occurs due to exposure to household substances especially in children is categorized under household poisons.
- More than 85% of household poisons occur in children during the period when substances are in use instead of storage.

- **Route of poisoning:** Inhalation, ingestion, skin contact.

Table 12.18

| | |
|---|---|
| **Medicines** | • If not kept out of reach of children or not taken as prescribed can prove toxic.<br>• Common cold, flu, analgesics account a large number of poisoning. |
| **Personal care products** | • Perfumes, nail removers, mouthwash, toothpaste are the common causes.<br>• These products are commonly involved in unintentional poisoning in children under the age of 6 years. |
| **Cleaning products** | • Bleach, ammonia, furniture polish, drain cleaners, oven cleaners, detergents, dishwashing powders or liquid, turpentine. |

| | |
|---|---|
| **Paints** | • Whether by fume inhalation, ingestion or lead poisoning paints and paint thinners are harmful.<br>• During use there should be proper ventilation and be kept out of children's reach. |
| **Pesticides** | • When pest treatment is done, be careful about the areas treated and the instructions labelled.<br>• Rodent poisons be kept away from children and never be placed in food storage areas. |
| **Small batteries** | • The size and chemical composition makes them dangerous.<br>• These are used in watches, hearing aids causing accidental poisoning and choking in children. |

Table 12.19

| | |
|---|---|
| **Signs and symptoms** | • Nausea, vomiting, convulsions, confusion, respiratory distress, abnormal skin colour. |
| **Treatment (first aid)** | • Decontamination of patient immediately done.<br>• Skin contact: wash with plenty of water.<br>• Gaseous poison: let the patient in open fresh air area.<br>• Ingestion: drink water for dilution.<br>• Ingestion of medication: emesis. |
| **Prevention** | • Store potentially poisonous products or medicines locked and out of children's reach.<br>• Never leave the substance un-attended when in use. |

## Multiple Choice Questions

**1. Which acid is also known as oil of vitriol?**

A. Carbolic acid B. Sulphuric acid

C. Oxalic acid D. Nitric acid

**2. Which acid acquires yellowish tinge on exposing to air?**

A. Hydrochloric acid B. Carbolic acid

C. Sulphuric acid D. Nitric acid

**3. Which of the following is an organic acid?**

A. Sulphuric acid B. Hydrochloric acid

C. Nitric acid D. Formic acid

**4. MgSO4 is used in treatment of which substance?**

A. Carbamate poisoning B. Aluminum phosphide

C. Kerosene D. Oxalic acid

**5. What is the fatal dose of Melathion?**

A. 60gm B. 50gm C. 20gm D. 70gm

**6. Which substance is also known as Soda lye?**

A. Sodium hydroxide B. Sulphuric acid

C. Nitric acid D. Oxalic acid

**7. Which acid is known as Red spirit of Nitre?**

A. Sulphuric acid B. Nitric acid

C. Formic acid D. Hydrochloric acid

**8. Chvostek's sign is found in which acid poisoning?**

A. Oxalic acid B. Hydrochloric acid

C. Formic acid D. Sulphuric acid

**9. What is the fatal dose of kerosene?**

A. 2ml B. 5ml C. 8ml D. 10ml

**10. What percent of carbon monoxide resembles the symptoms of alcohol intoxication?**

A. 10-20% B. 30-40% C. 40-50% D. 60-70%

**Answer key for MCQs:**

| | |
|---|---|
| 1 | B |
| 2 | A |
| 3 | D |
| 4 | B |
| 5 | A |

| | |
|---|---|
| 6 | A |
| 7 | B |
| 8 | A |
| 9 | D |
| 10 | C |

# Ch. 13
# Substances of abuse

### 13.1 Madya and Madatyaya, Alcoholism:

- ***Nirukti:***

  मद्यः = मद् धातु+ यत प्रत्यय

- ***Paribhasha:***

  बुद्धिं लुम्पति यद् द्रव्यं मदकारि तदुच्यते
  तमोगुणप्रधानं च यथा मद्यसुराऽदिकम् (शा. पू. ख.४/२१)

The drugs which are predominantly having Tamo guna will be called as Madakari.

- ***Madya Guna:***

  लघूष्णतीक्ष्णसूक्ष्माम्लव्यवाय्याशुगमेव च।
  रूक्षं विकाशि विशदं मद्यं दशगुणं स्मृतम् (च. चि. २४/३०)

Laghu: light
Ushna: warm
Tikshna: sharp
Sukshma: minute
Amla: sour
Vyavayi: pervading
Ashu: fast
Ruksha: dryness
Vikasi: dilate
Vishada: non slimy

- ***Madya Dosha:***

  यथोपेतं पुनर्मद्यं प्रसङ्गाद्येन पीयते।
  रूक्षव्यायामनित्येन विषवद्याति तस्य तत्।। (च. चि. २४/२८)

The people who indulge in dry foods and exercises daily may cause even more harm.

Table 13.1

| Madya guna | Oja guna |
|---|---|
| Laghu | Guru |
| Ushna | Shit |
| Tikshna | Madhur |
| Sukshma | Snigdha |
| Amla | Mrudu |
| Vyavayi | Prasad |
| Ashu | Sneha |
| Ruksha | Sthira |
| Vikasi | Slakshan |
| Vishad | Pichhila |

- ***Madya janita roga:***

  मद्ये मोहो भयं शोकः क्रोधो मृत्युश्च संश्रितः |
  सोन्मादमदमूर्च्छायाः सापस्मारापतानकाः || (च. चि. २४/५६)

Confusion, fear, grief, anger, death may occur due to intake of alcohol. Alongwith psychosis, intoxication, epilepsy.

- ***Mada Avastha:***

  ओजस्यविहते पूर्वो ह्रदि च प्रतिबोधिते |
  मध्यमो विहतेऽल्पे च विहते तूत्तमो मदः || (च. चि. २४/३७)

**Stage 1:** When Madya spreads to heart but doesnot cause disturbance of Ojas.

प्रहर्षणः प्रीतिकरः पानान्नगुणदर्शकः ।
वाद्यगीतप्रहासानां कथानां च प्रवर्तकः ॥ ४२ ॥
न च बुद्धिस्मृतिहरो विषयेषु न चाक्षमः ।
सुखनिद्राप्रबोधश्च प्रथमः सुखदो मदः ॥ (च. चि. २४/४२-४३)

Excitement, passion, increase in food intake, indulges in music and narrates stories, doesnot effect the intellect.

**Stage 2:** There is some amount of Oja disturbance.

मुहुः स्मृतिर्मुहुर्मोहो(ऽ)व्यक्ता सज्जति वाङ्मुहुः ।
युक्तायुक्तप्रलापश्च प्रचलायनमेव च ॥ ४४ ॥
स्थानपानान्नसाङ्कथ्ययोजना सविपर्यया ।
लिङ्गान्येतानि जानीयादाविष्टे मध्यमे मदे ॥
(च. चि. २४/४४–४५)

Memory is affected, confusion, indistinct speech, improper movements and body language.

**Stage 3:** There occurs major amount of Oja disturbance.

तृतीयं तु मदं प्राप्य भग्नदार्विव निष्क्रियः ।
मदमोहावृतमना जीवन्नपि मृतैः समः ॥ ४८ ॥
रमणीयान् स विषयान्न वेत्ति न सुहृज्जनम् ।
यदर्थं पीयते मद्यं रतिं तां च न विन्दति ॥ ४६ ॥
कार्याकार्यं सुखं दुःखं लोके यच्च हिताहितम् ।
यदवस्थो न ज़ानाति कोऽवस्थां तां व्रजेद्बुधः ॥ ५० ॥
स दूष्यः सर्वभूतानां निन्द्यश्चाग्राह्य एव च ।
व्यसनित्वादुदर्के च स दुःखं व्याधिमश्नुत ॥
(च. चि. २४/४८–५१)

The person becomes like a log of wood totally stiff. There occurs visual disturbance and intellectual confusion. Does not recognize his friends and family. He doesn’t recognize happiness or sadness and doesnot know what is good or bad for him.

- ***Yuktipurvak Madyapana:***

तेषां त्रिकाणामष्टानां योजना युक्तिरुच्यते।
यया युक्त्या पिबन्मद्यं मद्यदोषैर्न युज्यते।।६६।।
मद्यस्य च गुणान् सर्वान् यथोक्तान् स समश्नुते।
धर्मार्थयोरपीडायै नरः सत्त्वगुणोच्छ्रितः।। (च. चि. २४/६६–७०)

When alcohol is intaken after proper analysis it is called Yuktipurvak. The person with dominant Satva Guna when takes alcohol in a limited quantity, he does not get bad effects.

- ***Madyapana Ayoga:***

क्रोधिनोऽनुचिताः क्षीणाः परिश्रान्ता मदक्षताः।
स्वल्पेनापि मदं शीघ्रं यान्ति मद्येन मानवाः।।

Anger, ksheena, tired, affected by alcohol, hunger or thirst are affected heavily even on a small quantity consumption of alcohol.

- ***Madatyaya:***

शरीरदुःखं बलवत् सम्मोहो (१) हृदयव्यथा।
अरुचिः प्रतता तृष्णा ज्वरः शीतोष्णलक्षणः।।१०१।।
शिरःपार्श्वास्थिसन्धीनां विद्युत्तुल्या (३) च वेदना।
जायतेऽतिबला जृम्भा स्फुरणं वेपनं श्रमः ।।१०२।।
उरोविबन्धः कासश्च हिक्का श्वासः प्रजागरः।
शरीरकम्पः कर्णाक्षिमुखरोगस्त्रिकग्रहः।।१०३।।
छर्द्यतीसारहृल्लासा वातपित्तकफात्मकाः।
भ्रमः प्रलापो रूपाणामसतां चैव दर्शनम्।।१०४।।
तृणभस्मलतापर्णपांशुभिश्चावपूरणम्।
प्रधर्षणं विहङ्गैश्च भ्रान्तचेताः स मन्यते।।१०५।।
व्याकुलानामशस्तानां स्वप्नानां दर्शनानि च।
मदात्ययस्य रूपाणि सर्वाण्येतानि लक्षयेत्।।

(च. चि. २४/१०१–१०६)

Table 13.2

| शरीरदुःखं | Body pain |
|---|---|
| सम्मोह | Confusion |
| हृदयव्यथा | Cardiac pain |
| अरुचिः | Anorexia |
| तृष्णा | Thirst |
| शीतोष्णज्वरः | Cold and heat characteristic feature |
| शिरःपार्श्वास्थिसन्धीनां वेदना | Head, flanks, bones, joints pain |
| जृम्भा | Yawning |
| स्फुरणं | Throbbing pain |
| वेपनं | Tremors |
| श्रमः | Fatigue |
| उरोविबन्धः | Congestion in chest |
| कास | Cough |
| हिक्का | Hiccups |
| श्वासः | Asthma |
| प्रजागरः | Sleeplessness |
| शरीरकम्पः | Body tremors |
| कर्णाक्षिमुखरोग | Ear, eyes, mouth disease |
| छर्द्यतीसारहृल्लासा | Vomiting, diarrhoea, nausea |
| भ्रमः | Giddiness |
| प्रलाप | Delirium |
| रूपाणामसतां चैव दर्शनम् | Hallucinations |
| तृणभस्मलतापर्णपांशुभिश्चावपूरणम् | Covered by leaf, ash, grass, creeper |
| भ्रान्तचेताः | Visuals of fear |
| व्याकुलानामशस्तानां स्वप्नानां | Dreams are inauspicious |

- ***Vataja Madatyaya Hetu:***

  स्त्रीशोकभयभाराध्वकर्मभिर्योऽतिकर्शितः।
  रूक्षाल्पप्रमिताशी च यः पिबत्यतिमात्रया।।
  रूक्षं परिणतं मद्यं निशि निद्रां विहत्य च।
  करोति तस्य तच्छीघ्रं वातप्रायं मदात्ययम्।।
  (च. चि. २४/८६–६०)

- Excess sexual intercourse, fear, carrying heavy weights, excess emaciated, eating dry foods in less quantity.
- Eating dry food with older alcohols at night are main causative factors.

- ***Vataja Madatyaya Lakshana:***

  हिक्काश्वासशिरःकम्पपार्श्वशूलप्रजागरैः।
  विद्याद्बहुप्रलापस्य वातप्रायं मदात्ययम्।। (च. चि. २४/६१)

- Hiccups, coughing, breathing problem, tremors pain in flanks, Sleeplessness, excess speech.

- ***Vataja Madatyaya Chikitsa:***
  - Unctuous and sour soup of common quail, patridge, peacock
  - Wheat + varuni froath
  - Meat of fleshy animals with pepper + ginger +
  - Meat of animals + pomegranate juice
  - After food when thirsty take varuni froth, pomegranate juice, sour gruel, froth of curd
  - Hot bath
  - Shali rice
  - Massaging
  - Thick agaru paste
  - Strong Agaru essence
  - Affectionate hug from women with warmth of hips,

breast

- ○ Swaddling warmth of comfort home.

- ***Pittaja Madatyaya Hetu:***

  तीक्ष्णोष्णं मद्यमम्लं च योऽतिमात्रं निषेवते।
  अम्लोष्णतीक्ष्णभोजी च क्रोधनोऽग्न्यातपप्रियः।।
  तस्योपजायते पित्ताद्विशेषेण मदात्ययः।
  स तु वातोल्बणस्याशु प्रशमं याति हन्ति वा।।
  (च. चि. २४/६२–६३)

- Sharp, hot, sour alcohol in more quantity.
- Sour, hot, sharp food intake with exposure to anger, sun, fire.

- ***Pittaja Madatyaya Lakshana:***

  तृष्णादाहज्वरस्वेदमूर्च्छातीसारविभ्रमैः।
  विद्याद्धरितवर्णस्य पित्तप्रायं मदात्ययम।। (च. चि. २४/६४)

- Thirst, burning sensation, fever, sweating, unconsciousness, Giddiness, greenish discoloration.

- ***Pittaja Madatyaya Chikitsa:***
  - ○ Liquor made of mridvika, sharkara
  - ○ Parched grain flour + dates + grapes + pomegranate
  - ○ Goat meat prepared with pea + amalaka + dadima
  - ○ Induce complete emesis by water, liquor, grape juice
  - ○ When haemoptesis give decoction of guduchi + patola + devdaru
  - ○ Kola + dadima + vrikshamla paste apply inside of mouth to pacify thirst
  - ○ Cold water for drinking, bathing, shower

Cold exposure of moonlight

- Cold touch of linen

- Touch of women bathed with sandalwood
- Feel of lotus leaves, lily, sandal water

- ***Kaphaja Madatyaya Hetu:***

तरुणं मधुरप्रायं गौडं पैष्टिकमेव वा।
मधुरस्निग्धगुर्वाशी यः पिबत्यतिमात्रया ।।
अव्यायामदिवास्वप्नशय्यासनसुखे रतः।
मदात्ययं कफप्रायं स शीघ्रमधिगच्छति ।।
(च. चि. २४/६५–६६)

- Freshly made sweet, having jaggery and flour in excess.
- Intake of sweet, unctuous food with lack of exercise, day sleep, always being in comfort zone lying on bed.

- ***Kaphaja Madatyaya Lakshana:***

छर्द्यरोचकहृल्लासतन्द्रास्तैमित्यगौरवैः।
विद्याच्छीतपरीतस्य कफप्रायं मदात्ययम् ।। (च. चि. २४/६७)

- Vomiting, anorexia, nausea, laziness, feeling as if covered by wet cloth, heaviness.

- ***Kaphaja Madatyaya Chikitsa:***
- Water boiled with bala + kantakari
- Water boiled with musta pacifies all types of alcoholism
- Sour soup of amalaka with barley food
- Old arishta + sharkara + honey
- Meat roasted in earthen plate with sour and pungent substances with madya
- Jeerak + sauvarchal + twak + ela + amlavetas + marich + sugar clears all srotas
- Arid food
- Arid drinks
- Hot water bath

- Physical exercise

- ***Sannipataja Madatyaya Hetu:***

विषस्य ये गुणा दृष्टाः सन्निपातप्रकोपणाः।
त एव मद्ये दृश्यन्ते विषे तु बलवत्तराः।।
हन्त्याशु हि विषं किञ्चित् किञ्चिद्रोगाय कल्पते।
यथा विषं तथैवान्त्यो ज्ञेयो मद्यकृतो मदः।।
तस्मात् त्रिदोषजं लिङ्गं सर्वत्रापि मदात्यय।
दृश्यते रूपवैशेष्यात् पृथक्त्वं चास्य लक्ष्यते।।
(च. चि. २४/९८–१००)

**NOTE:**

- Harshana Chikitsa should be done in all madatyaya.
- Stay at cooling gardens, clean clothing, perfumes, garlands, laughter, singing.
- Milk may be administered in person with vata and pitta. It will increase strength and acts like a boon just like rains in extreme summer.

- ***Dhwansak and Vikshaya:***
- ध्वंसक लक्षणः

श्लेष्मप्रसेकः कण्ठास्यशोषः शब्दासहिष्णुता।
तन्द्रानिद्रातियोगश्च ज्ञेयं ध्वंसकलक्षणम्।। (च. चि. २४/२०१)

- Excess salivation, throat and mouth become dry, in-tolerance to sound.
- Laziness, sleepiness are in excess.

- विक्षय लक्षणः

हृत्कण्ठरोगः सम्मोहश्छर्दिरङ्गरुजा ज्वरः।
तृष्णा कासः शिरःशूलमेतद्विक्षयलक्षणम्।। (च. चि. २४/२०२)

- Diseases of heart and throat, confusion, vomiting, body pain, thirst, coughing, headache.

- ***Dhwansak and Vikshaya Chikitsa:***

  तयोः कर्म तदेवेष्टं वातिके यन्मदात्यय।
  तौ हि प्रक्षीणदेहस्य जायेते दुर्बलस्य वै।।
  बस्तयः सर्पिषः पानं प्रयोगः क्षीरसर्पिषोः।
  अभ्यङ्गोद्वर्तनस्नानान्यन्नपानं च वातनुत्।।
  ध्वंसको विक्षयश्चैव कर्मणाऽनेन शाम्यति।
  युक्तमद्यस्य मद्योत्थो न व्याधिरुपजायते।।
  (च. चि. २४/ २०३–२०५)

- The drinking disorders will never occur in person who follow proper method.
- In people suffering from disease should be given Basti, Ghritapana, milk with ghee, Abhyanga, Udvartana, food having properties of Vata shamana.

## 13.2 Addiction: Alcohol, Bhanga, Opioids, Tobacco and Digitalis.

### *1. Alcohol:*

Alcohol addiction (also called alcohol use disorder, or AUD) is a chronic disease characterized by an inability to control or stop drinking despite negative consequences to health, relationships, or work.

- Alcohol affects the brain's reward and pleasure centers by increasing dopamine and GABA activity. Over time:

a) The brain adapts to alcohol, leading to tolerance (needing more to feel the same effect).

b) When alcohol is reduced or stopped, withdrawal symptoms occur (anxiety, tremors, sweating, insomnia, seizures).

### *Signs and Symptoms:*

- **Physical:**
  - Tremors or shaking in the morning

- Sweating, nausea, poor appetite
- Memory loss or blackouts
- Liver issues (jaundice, pain, fatigue)

- **Behavioural:**
  - Craving alcohol regularly
  - Losing control over drinking
  - Neglecting work, family, or hygiene
  - Drinking alone or secretly
  - Continuing despite health or legal problems

- **Health effects:**
  - Chronic alcohol use can cause:
  - **Liver disease:** fatty liver, hepatitis, cirrhosis
  - **Heart disease:** high blood pressure, arrhythmias
  - **Brain damage:** memory issues, neuropathy
  - **Cancers:** mouth, throat, liver, breast

***Treatment Options:***

- Medical Detoxification: Supervised withdrawal to prevent complications (especially seizures or delirium tremens).

- **Psychotherapy:**
  - Cognitive Behavioral Therapy (CBT) to change drinking habits.
  - Motivational Enhancement Therapy to build motivation.
  - Family therapy and support systems.

- **Support Groups:**
  - Alcoholics Anonymous (AA) or local de-addiction groups.
  - Peer support and accountability.

- Lifestyle Changes:
  - Regular exercise, nutritious diet.
  - Stress management (yoga, meditation, hobbies).
  - Avoiding triggers (places, people, stressors associated with drinking).
  - **Medhya Rasayanas (brain tonics):** Brahmi, Shankhapushpi, Ashwagandha.
  - **Shodhana therapy (detox):** Panchakarma under supervision.
  - **Satvavajaya Chikitsa:** strengthening willpower and mind control.

***2. Bhanga:***

From a modern medical point of view, Bhanga addiction (addiction to cannabis or marijuana) is classified under Cannabis Use Disorder (CUD) — a condition recognized by the World Health Organization (WHO) and the Diagnostic and Statistical Manual of Mental Disorders (DSM-5).

Bhanga is prepared from the leaves and flowering tops of the Cannabis sativa plant.

The main psychoactive chemical is Δ9-tetrahydrocannabinol (THC), which acts on the brain's cannabinoid receptors and produces euphoria, relaxation, and altered perception.

**Mechanism of addiction:**

- THC affects the brain's endocannabinoid system, which regulates mood, memory, pain, and reward.
- THC binds to CB1 receptors in the brain.
- This releases dopamine (the "pleasure chemical"), producing a sense of relaxation or euphoria.
- With repeated use, the brain adapts — leading to tolerance (needing more to feel the same effect).
- When use stops, the person experiences withdrawal symptoms,

showing dependence.

**Signs and Symptoms:**
- Behavioral symptoms:
- Strong craving for Bhanga
- Inability to control or reduce use
- Neglect of work, study, or family duties
- Social withdrawal or isolation

**Physical symptoms:**
- Red eyes, dry mouth
- Increased appetite
- Impaired coordination and reaction time
- Irregular sleep pattern

**Psychological symptoms:**
- Euphoria and relaxation (initially)
- Memory loss, poor focus
- Anxiety, panic attacks
- Hallucinations or paranoia (high doses)
- Depression or lack of motivation (long-term use)

**Withdrawal symptoms:**
- Irritability and restlessness
- Anxiety and depression
- Difficulty sleeping (insomnia, vivid dreams)
- Loss of appetite
- Physical discomfort (headache, sweating, tremors)

**Health effects of long-term use:**
- *Brain and Mental Health:*
- Impaired memory and learning
- Decreased motivation (known as amotivational syndrome)
- Increased risk of psychosis in genetically vulnerable

individuals
- Worsening of anxiety or depression

**Respiratory Effects:**
- Chronic cough, bronchitis, lung irritation (if smoked).

**Reproductive Effects:**
- Reduced sperm count and motility in men.
- Menstrual irregularities in women.

**Treatment:**
- *Behavioral Therapies:*
- The cornerstone of treatment — since there is no specific medicine approved for cannabis addiction yet.
- Cognitive Behavioral Therapy (CBT): Helps change patterns of thought and behavior.
- Motivational Enhancement Therapy (MET): Builds motivation to quit.

**Rehabilitation Programs:**
- Outpatient counselling or inpatient de-addiction centres for severe cases
- Support groups (e.g., Marijuana Anonymous, 12-step programs)

**Lifestyle and Relapse Prevention**
- Regular physical exercise and meditation.
- Healthy diet and hydration.
- Avoid triggers (friends, locations, stressors).
- Develop new hobbies and social support.

***3. Opioids:***

Opioid addiction is a chronic, relapsing disorder characterized by compulsive drug seeking, continued use despite harmful consequences, and long-lasting changes in the brain. It involves dependence on opioids such as morphine, heroin, codeine, oxycodone, fentanyl, and methadone.

According to the World Health Organization (WHO), opioid dependence is "a cluster of behavioral, cognitive, and physiological phenomena that develop after repeated opioid use."

Opioids bind to mu, kappa, and delta receptors in the brain and spinal cord, reducing pain perception and creating a sense of euphoria.

Repeated exposure alters dopamine regulation in the mesolimbic reward pathway, leading to tolerance and physical dependence.

**Signs and Symptoms:**

***Physical Symptoms:***

- Pinpoint pupils
- Slurred speech
- Drowsiness or sedation
- Nausea, constipation
- Itching and sweating

***Psychological Symptoms:***

- Euphoria followed by apathy or irritability
- Anxiety or depression
- Craving and compulsive drug use

***Withdrawal Symptoms:***

- Muscle aches, restlessness, yawning
- Insomnia, diarrhoea, vomiting
- Gooseflesh skin ("cold turkey")

***Complications:***

- Overdose (can lead to respiratory depression and death)
- Infectious diseases (HIV, Hepatitis B/C due to needle sharing)

- Cognitive impairment
- Social and occupational dysfunction
- Legal and financial problems

**Management and Treatment:**

***Detoxification:***

- Gradual withdrawal under medical supervision using medications such as methadone or buprenorphine.

***Psychotherapy:***

- Cognitive Behavioral Therapy (CBT)
- Motivational Enhancement Therapy (MET)
- Family and group counseling
- Rehabilitation and Social Support:
- Community-based programs
- Support groups like Narcotics Anonymous (NA)

***Prevention:***

- Rational prescription of opioids
- Patient education on risks and alternatives
- Monitoring through prescription drug databases
- Early identification and intervention

***4. Tobacco:***

Tobacco addiction, also known as nicotine dependence, is a chronic relapsing condition characterized by compulsive use of tobacco products despite harmful consequences. It is one of the most common forms of substance addiction worldwide and a leading cause of preventable disease and death.

According to the World Health Organization (WHO), tobacco dependence is "a disorder of behavior, cognition, and physiology that develops after repeated tobacco use."

The addictive component of tobacco is nicotine, which stimulates the brain's reward pathways, leading to dependence.

**Forms of Tobacco Use:**

- Smoking forms: Cigarettes, bidis, cigars, pipes, hookah
- Smokeless forms: Chewing tobacco, gutkha, khaini, snuff, zarda, pan masala

**Causes and Risk Factors:**

- Nicotine's addictive nature: stimulates dopamine release in the brain
- Psychological factors: stress, anxiety, depression, low self-esteem
- Social and cultural influences: peer pressure, media exposure, family habits
- Early initiation: starting tobacco use at a young age increases dependence
- Genetic predisposition: family history of substance use

**Signs and Symptoms:**

***Physical Signs:***

- Persistent smoking or chewing habit
- Yellow-stained teeth and fingers
- Chronic cough, shortness of breath
- Halitosis (bad breath)

***Psychological Symptoms:***

- Craving for tobacco
- Anxiety or irritability when not using tobacco
- Difficulty concentrating

***Withdrawal Symptoms:***

- Headache, restlessness
- Fatigue and increased appetite
- Insomnia

- Depressed mood

**Complications:**

***Health Effects:***

- Cancer: Lung, oral, throat, esophagus, pancreas
- Cardiovascular: Hypertension, coronary heart disease, stroke
- Respiratory: Chronic bronchitis, COPD, emphysema
- Reproductive: Infertility, low birth weight in newborns

**Management and Treatment:**

***Behavioral Therapy:***

- Cognitive Behavioral Therapy (CBT)
- Motivational Interviewing
- Group or family counseling

***Pharmacotherapy:***

- Nicotine Replacement Therapy (NRT): gum, patch, lozenge, nasal spray
- Non-nicotine medications:
- Bupropion – reduces craving and withdrawal
- Varenicline – partial agonist at nicotine receptors

***Supportive Measures:***

- Stress reduction (yoga, meditation, physical activity)
- Self-help programs and helplines (e.g., WHO Quitline)
- Peer support groups

***Prevention:***

- Public health education campaigns
- School-based anti-tobacco programs
- Restriction of advertisement and sale
- Smoke-free environments
- Warning labels on tobacco product

### *5. Digitalis:*

Digitalis refers to a group of cardiac glycosides derived from the Digitalis purpurea (foxglove) plant. The main active compound is digoxin.

While digitalis is therapeutically used in heart failure and atrial fibrillation, prolonged or excessive use can lead to dependence and toxicity, sometimes referred to as digitalis addiction or digitalis habituation.

Digitalis addiction is a condition in which a person becomes dependent—physically or psychologically—on digitalis or its derivatives, often due to prolonged therapeutic use. It is characterized by a compulsive need to continue the drug despite toxic effects or lack of clinical indication.

**Causes and Risk Factors:**

- Prolonged medical use of digitalis for cardiac conditions
- Self-medication or dosage errors
- Elderly patients with reduced renal function (drug accumulates easily)
- Drug interactions (with diuretics, quinidine, verapamil, etc.)
- Psychological dependence due to perceived improvement in symptoms

**Signs and symptoms:**

***Gastrointestinal Symptoms:***

- Loss of appetite (anorexia)
- Nausea, vomiting, diarrhoea

***Neurological Symptoms:***

- Headache, dizziness
- Confusion, delirium, or hallucinations
- Visual disturbances (blurred vision, yellow or green halos around lights — "xanthopsia")

***Cardiac Manifestations:***

- Bradycardia
- Ventricular arrhythmias (e.g., PVCs, ventricular tachycardia)
- Heart block

***Psychological Features:***

- Anxiety or fear of missing the drug
- Emotional dependence on continued use

***Management:***

- Discontinuation of Digitalis:
- Stop or reduce the dose immediately under medical supervision.
- Monitor for withdrawal arrhythmias if the drug is stopped suddenly.
- Correction of Contributing Factors:
- Maintain normal potassium and magnesium levels
- Treat dehydration
- Supportive Care:
- ECG monitoring
- Hydration and electrolyte balance
- Psychological counselling if habitual misuse is present

***Prevention:***

- Careful dosing and monitoring in elderly and renal patients
- Regular measurement of serum digoxin levels
- Educating patients about toxicity symptoms
- Avoiding unnecessary long-term use
- Monitoring drug interactions

## 13.3 Drugs of abuse: Lysergic Acid Diethylamide and 3,4-methylenedioxymethamphetamine:

### *1. LSD:*

Lysergic Acid Diethylamide (LSD) is a potent hallucinogenic (psychedelic) drug derived from ergot alkaloids found in the fungus Claviceps purpurea.

LSD is known for its profound psychological effects, including altered perception, mood changes, and sensory distortions.

Although it does not typically cause physical dependence, it can lead to psychological addiction in some individuals due to its powerful mind-altering effects.

LSD addiction refers to a state of psychological dependence where a person feels a strong desire or compulsion to repeatedly use LSD to achieve euphoria, hallucinations, or altered consciousness, despite harmful psychological or social consequences.

**Chemical nature:**

- Full name: Lysergic Acid Diethylamide
- Class: Hallucinogen / Psychedelic
- Common street names: Acid, Blotter, Tabs, Lucy, Trips
- Usually taken orally on blotter paper, sugar cubes, or tablets

**Psychological Effects:**

- Visual and auditory hallucinations ("seeing colours," "hearing sounds")
- Distorted sense of time and space
- Euphoria or heightened emotional states
- Synesthesia (blending of senses)
- Mood swings, anxiety, or paranoia

**Physical Effects:**

- Dilated pupils

- Increased heart rate and blood pressure
- Tremors, sweating
- Dizziness, nausea

Tolerance: Develops rapidly after repeated use; larger doses are needed for the same effect.

Physical dependence: Minimal or absent — no classic withdrawal symptoms.

Psychological dependence: Strong; users may crave the experience or emotional escape LSD provides.

**Acute Reactions:**
- Intense fear, panic, confusion
- Paranoia, delusions, or psychotic behaviour
- Accidents or self-harm due to loss of judgment

**Chronic Effects:**
- Persistent psychosis (hallucinations or delusions lasting weeks or months)
- Hallucinogen Persisting Perception Disorder (HPPD): Flashbacks of visual disturbances even after cessation
- Anxiety, depression, depersonalization

**Social and Occupational Impact:**
- Poor academic/work performance
- Isolation, risky behaviours, or legal issues

**Management and Treatment:**

***Acute Intoxication:***
- Calm, quiet environment
- Reassurance and monitoring
- Benzodiazepines (e.g., diazepam) for severe anxiety or agitation

- Antipsychotics (e.g., haloperidol) for hallucinations or psychosis

***Long-Term Treatment:***

- Psychological counselling (Cognitive Behavioural Therapy, Motivational Therapy)
- Support groups and social rehabilitation
- Treatment of coexisting disorders (depression, anxiety, psychosis)
- No specific pharmacological antidote exists for LSD. Management is mainly supportive and psychotherapeutic.

***Prevention:***

- Health education about hallucinogen risks
- Early identification of users in schools/colleges
- Psychological support for stress and curiosity-driven use
- Legal restrictions and public awareness campaigns

***2. MDMA:***

(3,4-methylenedioxymethamphetamine), commonly known as Ecstasy or Molly, is a synthetic psychoactive drug that has both stimulant and hallucinogenic properties.

It is widely used as a "party drug" for its euphoric and energizing effects, but repeated use can lead to psychological dependence, neurotoxicity, and serious health complications.

MDMA addiction refers to a pattern of compulsive use of MDMA characterized by craving, loss of control, and continued use despite harmful physical, mental, or social consequences.

While physical dependence is mild, psychological addiction can be strong due to the drug's pleasurable effects on mood and perception.

**Effects of MDMA:**

***Short-term Effects:***

- Euphoria and heightened sensory perception
- Increased sociability and emotional closeness
- Enhanced energy and endurance
- Reduced fear and anxiety

***Physical Effects:***

- Increased heart rate and blood pressure
- Jaw clenching, teeth grinding (bruxism)
- Sweating, dehydration
- Nausea, blurred vision
- Hyperthermia (dangerous overheating)

***After effects:***

- Fatigue, depression
- Irritability, anxiety
- Sleep disturbance

***Dependence and Tolerance:***

- Tolerance: Develops rapidly; users need higher doses for the same effect.
- Psychological dependence: Strong — users crave the emotional high and social connectedness MDMA produces.
- Physical dependence: Mild; withdrawal symptoms are mostly emotional or behavioural rather than physical.

***Withdrawal Symptoms:***

- Fatigue and low mood
- Sleep problems
- Loss of appetite
- Irritability or anxiety
- Difficulty concentrating
- Intense craving for the drug

***Acute Complications:***

- Hyperthermia (can lead to organ failure)
- Dehydration or hyponatremia (from over drinking water)
- Cardiac arrhythmias or hypertension
- Serotonin syndrome (especially if combined with antidepressants)

***Chronic Complications:***

- Memory impairment and cognitive decline
- Depression, anxiety, or persistent mood changes
- Sleep disturbances
- Liver and kidney damage
- Psychological dependence and social dysfunction

**Management and Treatment:**

***Acute Intoxication:***

- Cool the body if hyper thermic
- Hydration with electrolyte balance
- Benzodiazepines (e.g., diazepam) for agitation or seizures
- Treat complications like rhabdomyolysis or hyponatremia

***Long-Term Treatment:***

- Psychotherapy:
- Cognitive Behavioural Therapy (CBT)
- Motivational Enhancement Therapy (MET)
- Group or family counselling

***Rehabilitation programs:***

- Support groups and relapse-prevention education
- Stress management (yoga, meditation, exercise)

***Prevention:***

- School and community-based education about MDMA risks
- Regulation and monitoring of rave or club drug use

- Early psychological counselling for high-risk youth
- Public awareness campaigns about synthetic drug dangers

**13.4 Narcotic Drugs and Psychotropic Substances Act (NDPS):** The Narcotic Drugs and Psychotropic Substances Act (NDPS Act) was enacted by the Government of India in 1985 to control and regulate the operations relating to narcotic drugs and psychotropic substances.

It aims to prevent drug abuse and illicit trafficking, while allowing legitimate medical and scientific use.

To control, regulate, and prohibit the production, manufacture, possession, sale, purchase, transport, and consumption of narcotic drugs and psychotropic substances.

To ensure that narcotic and psychotropic substances are available for medical and scientific purposes only.

To prevent misuse and illegal trafficking of such substances.

To provide stringent punishment for offenders.

***Structure of the NDPS Act:***

I. Preliminary (definitions, scope)
II. Authorities and Officers (Narcotics Control Bureau, etc.)
III. Prohibition, control, and regulation of operations
IV. Offences and Penalties
V. Procedure and Miscellaneous provisions

***Regulatory Authorities:***

- Narcotics Control Bureau (NCB) – established in 1986 under Section 4(3) of the NDPS Act.
- Main agency responsible for coordination and enforcement.
- Works under the Ministry of Home Affairs.
- State and Central Governments – empowered to frame rules

for control and monitoring.

**Important Provisions:**

***Cultivation and Production:***

- Cultivation of coca, opium poppy, or cannabis requires special license from the government.
- Unauthorized cultivation or production is punishable under the Act.

***Possession and Consumption:***

- Possession, sale, or use of narcotic or psychotropic substances without authorization is prohibited.

***Punishments:***

- Small quantity   Up to the limit specified by government: Up to 1 year imprisonment or fine up to Rs.10,000, or both
- More than small but less than commercial quantity: Up to 10 years imprisonment and fine up to Rs.1 lakh
- Commercial quantity   Above government-specified limit 10 to 20 years imprisonment and fine Rs.1–2 lakh (extendable)

***Amendments:***

- 1989 Amendment: Introduced stricter punishment and bail restrictions.
- 2001 Amendment: Introduced quantity-based punishment (small, intermediate, commercial).
- 2014 Amendment: Allowed medical and scientific use of essential narcotic drugs (e.g., morphine) under simplified procedures.

***Rehabilitation and Treatment (Section 64A):***

- Provides immunity from prosecution to addicts who voluntarily seek treatment from government-approved centres.
- Emphasis on rehabilitation over punishment for first-time

users seeking help.

***Role of the NDPS Act in Public Health:***

- Controls misuse of prescription opioids, sedatives, and stimulants.
- Enables safe use of narcotics in palliative care, anesthesia, and pain management.
- Promotes coordination between law enforcement and health agencies.

**Multiple Choice Questions**

**1. Which of the following is Madya Guna?**

A. Guru B. Shit C. Madhura D. Amla

**2. How many chapters are there in NDPS act?**

A. 2 B. 5 C. 10 D. 13

**3. Digoxin active compound is found in?**

A. Digitalis B. Tobacco C. Opioids D. None

**4. NDPS act was enacted in?**

A. 1895 B. 1985 C. 2000 D. 1900

**5.**छर्द्यरोचकहृल्लासतन्द्रास्तैमित्यगौरवैः **lakshana of which Madatyaya?**

A. Kaphaja B. Pittaja C. Vataja D. Sannipataja

**6.** अम्लोष्णतीक्ष्णभोजी च क्रोधनोऽग्न्यातपप्रियः **indicates hetu of which Madatyaya?**

A. Sannipataja B. Pittaja C. Kaphaja D. Vataja

**7. Which of the following is derived from ergot alkaloids?**

A. Tobacco B. LSD C. Opioids D. None

**8. Which substance is commonly known as Molly?**
A. MDMA B. Tobacco C. LSD D. Bhanga

**9. What is derived from foxglove plant?**
A. Bhanga B. Digitalis C. Opioids D. Tobacco

**10.**हिक्काश्वासशिरःकम्पपार्श्वशूलप्रजागरैः **indicates which Madatyaya?**
A. Vataja B. Pittaja C. Kaphaja D. Sannipataja

**Answer key for MCQs:**

| 1 | D |
|---|---|
| 2 | B |
| 3 | A |
| 4 | B |
| 5 | A |

| 6 | B |
|---|---|
| 7 | B |
| 8 | A |
| 9 | B |
| 10 | A |

# Ch. 14
# Agada tantra Perspectives on Cancer

## 14.1 Toxic carcinogens:

***A: Cancers and Carcinogens:***

- Cancer is the leading cause of death in 21st Century. In Ayurveda, it is mentioned as Arbuda.
- Carcinogens cause damage to DNA and causes alters in functions or mutations are caused.
- Carcinogens steadily build up in body and causes cancer.

- Contact with carcinogens:
    - Lifestyle habits like tobacco chewing, smoking, drinking alcohol.
    - Exposure to carcinogens at work place.
    - Viruses like HPV causes cancer.
    - 5%-12% are inherited mutations causing cancer. When such people are exposed to carcinogens, are at higher risk of cancer occurrence.

***Common carcinogens:***

- **Age:** Although people of any age can get it. But older people are more at risk.
- **Genetics:** Family history may put more risk of cancer. An ancestor with a type of cancer increases the progeny risk to have that cancer.
- **Radon:** It is present in safe amount in environment. But when it builds up indoor and is inhaled, causes damage to the lining of lungs.

- **Tobacco:** There are 70 chemicals in tobacco known to cause cancer. Smoking is also harmful whether it is active or passive smoking.
- **Asbestos:** Tiny fibers in asbestos helps to strengthen ceilings, tiles, car parts. When these fibers break down causes build up in lungs, increasing risk for cancer.
- **Formaldehyde:** It is present in some plywood and household products. Studies have shown it is known for its harmful effects causing cancer.
- **UV rays:** When exposed to sun or tanning bed, rays get absorbed in skin and causes cell damage leading to skin cancer. Pollution and climate changes have made the rays exposure even stronger leading to increased chances of cancer.
- **Alcohol:** There are increasing odds of cancer for alcohol consumers. Cancers of Head and neck, esophagus, breast, liver, colorectal.
- **Processed meat:** Bacon, salami, pepperoni, sausage which may be preserved or flavored causes an increased chance of colon cancer.
- **Engine exhaust:** Trucks, bus, cars and even train engines run on diesel which release gas and soot. These are considered to cause lung cancer.
- **Gasoline:** as it contains aromatics.
- **Alkylating Anti-neoplastic Agents:** Mechlorethamine.
- **Low refining or unrefined mineral oils.**
- **Alkylating agents:** Dimethyl sulfate.

Table 14.1 Toxic carcinogens

| Carcinogen | Occupational sources | Associated cancer site |
|---|---|---|
| Arsenic and it's compounds | • Alloys, smelting byproduct.<br>• Semiconductor devices, herbicide, fungicide.<br>• Medications like melarsoprol. | • Lung, skin.<br>• Hemangiosarcoma. |
| Asbestos | • Roofing papers, floor tiles.<br>• Fire resistant textiles, friction linings like brake pads. | • Asbestosis<br>• Pleural mesothelioma, peritoneal mesothelioma. |
| Benzene | • Light fuel oil, solvent commodity chemical. | • Leukemia, Hodgkin's lymphoma. |
| Beryllium and it's compounds | • Aerospace application, nuclear reactors. | • Lung cancer. |
| Cadmium and it's compounds | • Yellow pigments, solders batteries.<br>• Metal paintings and coatings. | • Prostate cancer. |
| Hexavalent chromium compounds | • Paints, pigments, preservation. | • Lung cancer. |
| Vinyl chloride | • Product of poly-vinyl chloride. | • Hemangiosarcoma<br>• Liver cancer. |
| Radium-224, Radium-226, Plutonium-238 | • Nuclear fuel processing | • -Bone are involved |

***B. Arbuda:***

- **Nidan and Samprapti:**

सम्मूर्च्छिता मांसमभिप्रदूष्य।
वृत्तं स्थिरं मन्दरुजं महान्तमनल्पमूलं चिरवृद्ध्यपाकम् ।।
कुर्वन्ति मांसोपचयं तु शोफं तमर्बुदं शास्त्रविदो वदन्ति।
(सु.नि.११/१३–१४))

Dosha aggravation causes muscle tissue causing muscle growth which is round, immovable slight pain, deep rooted, growing slowly causing Arbuda.

- **Bheda:**
    - **Acharya Charaka:** Vataja, Pittaja, Kaphaja, Medaja, Siraja, Mamsaja.
    - **Acharya Sushruta:** Vataja, Pittaja, Kaphaja, Raktaja,Mamsaja, Medoja.

- **Raktarbuda:**

दोषः प्रदुष्टो रुधिरं सिरास्तु सम्पीड्य सङ्कोच्य गतस्त्वपाकम्।।
सास्रावमुन्नह्यति मांसपिण्डं मांसाङ्कुरैराचितमाशुवृद्धिम्।
स्रवत्यजस्रं रुधिरं प्रदुष्टमसाध्यमेतद्रुधिरात्मकं स्यात्।।
रक्तक्षयोपद्रवपीडितत्वात् पाण्डुर्भवेत् सोऽर्बुदपीडितस्तु।
(सु.नि. ११/१५–१७)

Aggravated Dosha gets combined with blood in blood vessels. Causes squeezing and contraction in blood vessels. There occurs a growth of muscle with sprouts of muscle and increases in size quickly causing oozing of visited blood. Due to this person suffers from secondary disease Pandu Roga.

- **Mamsarbuda:**

मुष्टिप्रहारादिभिरर्दितेऽङ्गे मांसं प्रदुष्टं प्रकरोति शोफम्।।
अवेदनं स्निग्धमनन्यवर्णमपाकमश्मोपममप्रचाल्यम्।
प्रदुष्टमांसस्य नरस्य बाढमेतद्भवेन्मांसपरायणस्य।।
मांसार्बुदं त्वेतदसाध्यमुक्तं...। (सु.नि.११/१७–१८)

When there occurs injury to body by hit of fist, there occurs swelling which is painless, unctuous, same color as body, not forming pus, immovable. This occurs in person with excess intake of meat.

- **Arbuda Apaka Karan:**

न पाकमायान्ति कफाधिकत्वान्मेदोबहुत्वाच्च विशेषतस्तु।
दोषस्थिरत्वाद्ग्रथनाच्च तेषां सर्वार्बुदान्येव निसर्गतस्तु।।
(सु.नि.११/२२)

All Arbuda don't form pus, especially which are predominant in Kapha and Meda. This forms a hard lump.

- **Sadhya – Asadhyata:**

साध्यः: Vataja, Pittaja, Kaphaja, Medoja.
असाध्य: Raktaja, Mamsaja, Marma-sthana, Achala Arbuda.

- **Vataja Arbuda Chikitsa:**
  - Apply warm poultice application prepared with Karkaruka, Evaruka, Narikela, Priyala.
  - Administer Nadi Sweda.
  - Do Raktamokshana using Shrunga.
  - Patient be made drink Trivrit Sneha which should be cooked 100 times using Vata mitigating drugs. This should be added with milk and sour substances.

- **Pittaja Arbuda Chikitsa:**
  - Swedana be done with Pittaghna Dravya.
  - Warm poultice be applied and Virechana be given.
  - The tumor be rubbed with Udumbara, Shaka, Go-jihva.
  - Later, apply paste of Sarjarasa, Priyangu, Rodhra, Aragwadha, Soma be added with honey.
  - Ghrita prepared with Shyama, Girihva, Anjalaki, Saptalika.

- **Kaphaja Arbuda Chikitsa:**
  - Vamana be done, Raktamokshana be done.
  - Warm poultice prepared with excreta of dove and

pigeon, Kamsya, Shukla-neela, Langlaka.
  - Root of Kakadani and Gomutra be applied on the tumor.

- **Kshara Prayoga:**
  - Apply Kshara on the site and then Shastra should be used without harming the strength of patient.
  - Decoction prepared from leaves of Asphota, Jati, Karveera be used to clean the surface.
  - Later oil boiled with Vidanga, Patha, Triphala be used for healing.

- **Medo Arbuda Chikitsa:**
  - Initially fomentation be done, then cut open and remove the vitiated blood and be sutures quickly.
  - Later the wound be sprinkled with powder of Haridra, Grahadhuma, Rodhra, Manashila, Ela.
  - Later Karanja Taila be mixed with honey and be applied to cleanse the wound.

## 14.2 Toxicities due to chemotherapy & radiotherapy with its Ayurvedic approach:

- According to the modern therapy, chemo and radiotherapy are the treatment for cancerous cells.
- But these are highly toxic which damage healthy cells in the surrounding along with the cancerous cells.
- The side effects of the therapy may be acute, intermediate or late.

Table 14.2 Side effects

| Chemotherapy | Radiotherapy | Late complications |
|---|---|---|
| • Nausea, vomiting, diarrhea.<br>• Mucositis, alopecia, constipation. | • Fatigue, anorexia, nausea, vomiting.<br>• Altered taste sensation, sleep disturbance, headache, anemia, dry skin, constipation. | • Pharyngitis, esophagitis, laryngitis.<br>• Persistent dysphagia, fatigue, hepatotoxicity, infertility. |

- When the above side effects are looked upon, they show an aggravation of Pitta Dosha umder the disorders like Raktapitta, Raktadushti.
- Ayurvedic approach which may act as adjuvant therapy to chemo and be useful to give patient a good quality of life.

***Herbs help total healing, side effects and complications:***

- Kalmegh (Andrographis peniculata), Bhumyamlaki (Phyllanthus niruri), Pippali (Piper longum), Giriparpati (Podophyllum haxandrum), Guduchi (Tinospora cordifolia), Madhupushpa (Madhuca indica), Mulaka (Raphanus sativus).

***Herbal preparation for chemotherapy rehabilitation:***

- Pippali (Piper longum), Tulsi (Ocimum sanctum), Brahmi (Bacopa monieri), Guggulu (Commiphora wightii), Turmeric (Curcuma longa), Amalaki (Emblica officinalis).

***Use of Basti:***

- Basti Dravya and it's effects lowers the risk of adverse effects of chemotherapy.
- Chemotherapy stimulates melanocortin system in hypothalamus leading to anorexia.
- The drugs used in Basti regulates the normal functions of brain.
-

### 14.3 Agada and Visha Dravya Prayoga in prevention and management of cancer:

- Bilvadi Agada: Hepato-protective and Radio-toxicity protection.
- Kalyanaka Agada: Hepato-protective.
- Ajitagada: Nephron toxicity protective.
- Malatyaadi Agada: Haemo-toxicity protective.
- Dooshivishari Agada: Protects against Lichen planus.
- Bhunimbadi Agada: Protects against E.coli, Staphylococcus aureus, Shigella sonnei, Salmonella enterica.
- Vishaghna Mahakashaya: Protects against all types of cancer.
- Ayurvedic management: Snehana, Swedana, Vamana, Virechana, Basti, Nasya, Raktamokshana, Shirodhara.

**Multiple Choice Questions**

**1. Arsenic is found in which of the following?**

A. Paint B. Pigments C. Preservatives D. Fungicide

**2. Which of the following is not असाध्यArbuda?**

A. Raktaja B. Mamsaja C. Medoja D. Achala Arbuda

**3.** मुष्टिप्रहारादिभिरर्दितेऽङ्गे मांसं प्रदुष्टं प्रकरोति शोफम् || **indicates which type of Arbuda?**

A. Vataja B. Pittaja C. Mamsarbuda D. Raktarbuda

**4. Cadmium and it's compounds cause which type of cancer?**

A. Lung B. Prostate C. Liver D. Hemangiosarcoma

**5. Arsenic and it's compounds causes which cancer?**

A. Hemangiosarcoma B. Pleural mesothelioma
C. Prostate cancer D. Hodgkin's lymphoma

**6. Which of the following is a late complication of radiotherapy?**

A. Headache B. Alopecia C. Pharyngitis D. Constipation

**7. Phyllanthus niruri is the Latin name of?**

A. Guduchi B. Pippali C. Mulaka D. Bhumyamlaki

**8. Andrographis peniculata is the Latin name of?**

A. Mulaka B. Kalmegha C. Giriparpati D. Madhupushpa

**9. Which Arbuda Chikitsa has shown sprinkling Grahadhuma on wound?**

A. Medoja B. Pittaja C. Mamsaja D. Raktaja

**10. Which Arbuda Chikitsa shows rubbing of tumor with Go-jihva?**

A. Vataja B. Pittaja C. Kaphaja D. Mamsaja

**Answer key for MCQs:**

| | | | |
|---|---|---|---|
| 1 | D | 6 | C |
| 2 | C | 7 | D |
| 3 | C | 8 | B |
| 4 | B | 9 | A |
| 5 | A | 10 | B |

# Ch. 15

# Forensic Medicine (Vyavahara Ayurveda) and Medical Jurisprudence (Vidhi Vaidyaka)

## 15.1 Forensic medicine and Medical jurisprudence

- ***Definition of Forensic medicine:***
    - Latin word: Forum = legal and Medicine = medical aspect.
    - Branch of medicine which deals with the knowledge of medicine foe the purpose of law.
    - Deals with the application of medical knowledge to provide justice.

- ***Medical jurisprudence:***
    - Latin word: Juris = Law and Prudential = legal aspect of medical practice.
    - It mainly deals with the legal responsibilities of the physician.

- ***History of Vyavahara Ayurveda and Vidhivaidyaka:***

1. Code of Hummurabi of Babylon (2000-1000 BC): Oldest medico-legal code given by king of Babylon which deals with punishment for giving improper treatment.
2. Code of Hittite (1400 BC): Deals with providing compensation for improper treatment.
3. Roman law (451 BC): Deals with medico-legal aspects.
4. Hippocrates (460-377 BC): Describes about medical ethics, death and lethality of wound.
5. Justinian code (AD 529-564): Penalties for medical practice and principles of regulation of medical profession.
6. The Barbarian statute: Role of medical practitioner in

evaluation of injuries.

7. Forensic medicine in India:

- In India, King Manu gave various laws in his treatise Manusmruti.
- For various offenses like adultery, incest, unnatural sexual offense, seduction. Intoxication, illness and age, mental illness were also described.
- Charaka Samhita written by Agnivesha is the oldest treatise in $7^{th}$ Century BC. It describes regarding training, duties, privileges and social status of physician. It can be considered as the origin of medical ethics.
- Sushruta Samhita has described chapters concerning forensic science.
- In $4^{th}$ and $3^{rd}$ Century BC, Kautilya gave the law code, penal laws, medical practice regulations and medical knowledge for the purposes of law.

## 15.2 Introduction to Indian Penal Code, Indian Evidence Act and Criminal Procedure Code

- ***Indian Penal Code:***
    - It deals with substantial Criminal laws of India. It describes punishment for various criminal offense.

### *A. Criminal responsibility:*

Table 15.1

| | |
|---|---|
| 82 IPC | • A child under the age of 7 seven years is not capable of committing an offense. |
| 83 IPC | • A child of 7-12 years is capable of committing offense if he has attained enough maturity and can judge the nature consequences of his conduct. |
| 84 IPC | • Act of a person with an unsound mind is not an offense. It is related to insanity and criminal responsibility.<br>• MC Naughten Rule is a legal test for the criminal responsibility of insane under section 84 IPC. |

| | |
|---|---|
| 85 & 86 IPC | • As per 85 IPC, Act of an intoxicated person is not an offense, if he is intoxicated against his will.<br>• As per 86 IPC, Act of intoxicated person is an offense if he had the intention or knowledge of committing a crime. So the person is criminally responsible.<br>• These sections are related to drunkenness and criminal responsibility. |
| 87 IPC | • A person below 18 years of age cannot give a valid consent to suffer death or grievous hurt. |
| 88 IPC | • Act not intended for death, but can cause death or grievous hurt, done by consent and for the benefit of that person.<br>• Eg: Death of a patient caused by surgery by a surgeon. |
| 89 IPC | • A child under 12 years of age cannot give valid consent to suffer any harm which can occur from an act done in good faith for the benefit of a child.<br>• Eg: Consent for surgery. Only a guardian can give such consent. |
| 94 IPC | • Act to which a person is compelled by threat, is not an offense. |

### *B. Offenses related to criminal abortion and child birth:*

Table 15.2

| | |
|---|---|
| 312, 313, 314, 315 IPC | • For causing criminal abortion |
| 312 IPC | • Causing miscarriage with the consent of woman. (3 years of imprisonment +/- fine). |
| 313 IPC | • Causing miscarriage without the consent of lady. ( 10 years of imprisonment which can extend to life +/- fine). |
| 314 IPC | • Death of patient caused by miscarriage. (10 years of imprisonment +/- fine). |
| 315 IPC | • Act done to prevent the child being born alive or to cause to die if alive after birth. (10 years of imprisonment +/- fine). |

| | |
|---|---|
| 318 IPC | • Concealment of birth by secret disposal of dead body. (2 years of imprisonment +/- fine). |

### *C. Offenses affecting life:*

Table 15.3

| | |
|---|---|
| 299 IPC | • Culpable homicide not amounting to murder, causing death without the intention of causing death. |
| 300 IPC | • Murder (defining murder). |
| 301 IPC | • Culpable homicide causing death of the person other than the person who's death was intended. |
| 302 IPC | • Punishment of murder (death of life imprisonment). |
| 303 IPC | • Punishment of murder of life convict. |
| 304 IPC | • Punishment of culpable homicide, not amounting to murder (10 years of imprisonment +/- fine). |
| 305 IPC | • Abetment of suicide of child or insane person. |
| 306 IPC | • Abetment of suicide. |
| 307 IPC | • Attempt to murder (10 years of imprisonment +/- fine). |
| 308 IPC | • Attempt to commit culpable homicide (3-7 years imprisonment +/- fine). |
| 309 IPC | • Attempt to commit suicide (1 year of imprisonment + fine). |

### *D. Offenses related to hurt:*

Table 15.4

| | |
|---|---|
| 319 IPC | • Defines hurt. |
| 320 IPC | • Defines grievous hurt. |
| 321 IPC | • Voluntarily causing hurt. |
| 322 IPC | • Voluntarily causing grievous hurt. |
| 323 IPC | • Punishment for voluntarily causing hurt ( no provocation or dangerous weapon) (1 year of imprisonment). |
| 324 IPC | • Punishment of voluntarily causing hurt by dangerous weapon (3 years imprisonment +/- fine). |

| 325 IPC | • Punishment for voluntarily causing grievous hurt ( no provocation or dangerous weapon) (7 years of imprisonment +/- fine). |
|---|---|
| 326 IPC | • Voluntarily causing grievous hurt by dangerous weapon (10 years of imprisonment +/- fine). |
| 327 IPC | • Causing hurt to extort property (10 years of imprisonment +/- fine). |
| 328 IPC | • Causing hurt by poison (10 years of imprisonment +/- fine). |
| 329 IPC | • Causing grievous hurt to extort property (10 years imprisonment which can extend up to life +/- fine). |
| 331 IPC | • Causing grievous hurt to extort confession (10 years imprisonment +/- fine). |
| 332 IPC | • Causing grievous hurt to deter public servant from his duty (3 years imprisonment +/- fine). |
| 333 IPC | • Voluntarily causing grievous hurt to deter public servant while they are discharging the duty (10 years imprisonment +/- fine). |
| 334 IPC | • Causing hurt on provocation (1 month imprisonment +/- fine). |
| 335 IPC | • Causing grievous hurt on provocation (4 years imprisonment +/- fine). |
| 336 IPC | • Act endangering life or personal safety. |
| 337 IPC | • Causing hurt by endangering life or safety. |
| 338 IPC | • Causing grievous hurt by endangering life. |

***E. Offenses related to dowry:***

Table 15.5

| 304 – B IPC | • Dowry death ( 10 years of imprisonment which can extend up to life). |
|---|---|
| 498 – A IPC | • Punishment for cruelty by husband or his relatives. |

*F. Rape & other sexual offenses and assault:*

Table 15.6

| | |
|---|---|
| 228 IPC | • Prohibits the disclosure of identity of rape victim. |
| 375 IPC | • Defining rape. |
| 376 – A IPC | • Punishment for rape ( life imprisonment +/- fine). |
| 377 IPC | • Unnatural sexual offenses (10 years to life imprisonment +/- fine). |
| 354 IPC | • Assault or criminal force to woman with an intent to outrage her modesty. |
| 366 – A IPC | • Procuration of minor girl for illicit intercourse. |
| 351 IPC | • Defines assault. |
| 352-358 IPC | • Punishment for causing assault. |
| 509 IPC | • Word, gesture or intent to insult the modesty of a woman. |

*G. Perjury, hostile witness and false certificate:*

Table 15.7

| | |
|---|---|
| 191 IPC | • Giving false evidence (perjury under oath and hostile witness). |
| 192 IPC | • Fabricating false evidence (perjury). |
| 193 IPC | • Punishment for false evidence ( 7 years of imprisonment +/- fine). |
| 194 IPC | • Giving false evidence to procure conviction of capital offense. |
| 195 IPC | • Giving false evidence to procure conviction of offense punishable with imprisonment for life. |
| 197 IPC | • Issuing false certificate by a doctor is a criminal offense. |
| 201 IPC | • Causing disappearance of evidence. |
| (H) Others | |
| 304 – A IPC | • Causing death by negligence, which also includes medical negligence (2 years punishment or fine or both). |

| 53 IPC | • An accused can be examined by a medical practitioner at request of police, even without his consent or by force. |
|---|---|
| 330, 331 339, 341 IPCs | • Torture. |
| 361-369 IPCs | • Kidnapping. |
| 87-93 IPCs | • Legal protection to medical doctors. |
| 190 IPC | • Threat of refraining a person from applying protection to a public servant. |
| 201 IPC | • Punishment for embalming before autopsy. |

- **Indian Evidence Act - IEA (1872):**
    - This act was originally passed in British Raj in 1872.
    - It deals with the law of evidence and applies to all judicial proceedings in any court.
    - It is common to both criminal and civil procedure.

Table 15.8

| Part 1 | Chapter 1: Introduction of this act.<br>Chapter 2: Relevancy of the facts. |
|---|---|
| Part 2 | Chapter 3: Facts which need to be proved.<br>Chapter 4: Oral evidence.<br>Chapter 5: Documentary evidence.<br>Chapter 6: Circumstances when documentary evidence is given more importance than Oral evidence. |
| Part 3 | Chapter 7: Burden of proof.<br>Chapter 8: Estoppel.<br>Chapter 9: Witness.<br>Chapter 10: Improper admission and rejection of evidence. |

- **Criminal Procedure Code – CrPC (1973):**
    - It provides mechanism of punishment of offenses against substantive criminal law.

Table 15.9

| | |
|---|---|
| 2 ( C) CrPC | • Cognisable offense. |
| 6 – 25 CrPC | • Constitution of criminal courts and officer. |
| 26 CrPC | • Division offenses. |
| 27 – 35 CrPC | • Power of court. |
| 39 CrPC | • Every person should give information to nearest magistrate or police officer. If that person is away commission of or intention of commission of an offense which is punishable under IPC. |
| 40 CrPC | • Duty of officers appointed and every person residing in a village to inform unnatural death of the dead body found. |
| 160 CrPC | • Police officer has the power to summon any witness to police station for recording of statement (a male below 15 years and a woman cannot be called to police station). |
| 161 CrPC | • Police has the power to examine witness. |
| 162 CrPC | • Oral statements made to the police and recorded by the police should be signed. |
| 174 CrPC | • Police inquest. |
| 174 (3) CrPC | • Procedure in dowry death. |
| 175 CrPC | • Power of police to summon panchas. |
| 176 CrPC | • Magistrate inquest. |
| 225-237 CrPC | • Session's trial. |
| 238-265 CrPC | • Magistrate's trial. |
| Section 416 CrPC | • Postponement of capital sentences on pregnant woman or it's communication for imprisonment for life can be done by the high court. |
| Section 409 CrPC | • Withdrawal of cases and appeals by Sessions judge. |
| Section 410 CrPC | • Withdrawal of cases by Judicial magistrate. |

| | |
|---|---|
| Section 411 CrPC | • Making over or withdrawal of cases by executive magistrate. |
| Section 412 CrPC | • Reasons to be recorded: A sessions judge or magistrate making an order under Section – 408, 409, 410 or 411 shall record his reasons for making it. |

**Multiple Choice Questions**

**1. In which year was the Roman law passed?**

A. 461BC B. 377BC C. 451BC D. 529BC

**2. Which Samhita has described chapters regarding forensic medicine?**

A. Madhava nidana B. Sushruta samhita
C. Ashtanga sangraha D. Charaka Samhita

**3. Causing miscarriage with the consent of woman has imprisonment of how many years?**

A. 5 years B. 3 years C. 8 years D. 10 years

**4. Attempt to murder comes under which section of IPC?**

A. 302 B. 303 C. 306 D. 307

**5. Causing grievous hurt to extort confession comes under which section of IPC?**

A. 331 B. 332 C. 333 D. 334

**6. 304 – B of IPC is related to which offense?**

A. Hurt B. Dowry
C. Hostile witness D. Criminal responsibility

**7. 85 & 86 IPC is related to which offense?**

A. Perjury B. Criminal responsibility
C. Dowry D. False certificate

**8. Magistrate's trial comes under which section of CrPC?**

A. 160 B. 174 (3) C. 225-237 D. 238-265

**9. Indian Evidence Act was passed in which year?**

A. 1973 B. 1760 C. 1872 D. 1900

**10. Procuration of minor girl for illicit intercourse comes under which section of IPC?**

A. 366(A) B. 376(A) C. 356(A) D. 326(A)

**Answer key for MCQs:**

| | |
|---|---|
| 1 | C |
| 2 | B |
| 3 | B |
| 4 | D |
| 5 | A |

| | |
|---|---|
| 6 | B |
| 7 | B |
| 8 | D |
| 9 | C |
| 10 | A |

# Ch. 16

# Vaidya Sadvritta – Duties and Responsibilities of Medical Practitioner

## 16.1 Vaidya Sadvritta, medical ethics & code of conduct, Charaka oath and Hippocratic oath:

- ***Vaidya Guna (Qualities of a physician):***

  श्रुते पर्यवदातत्वं बहुशो दृष्टकर्मता।
  दाक्ष्यं शौचमिति ज्ञेयं वैद्ये गुणचतुष्टयम्।। (च.सू. ९/६)

- The physician should have sound knowledge of all the health literatures.
- Should have extensive practical knowledge and practice.
- Dexterity and cleanliness of body & mind are important

  विद्या वितर्को विज्ञानं स्मृतिस्तत्परता क्रिया।
  यस्यैते षड्गुणास्तस्य न साध्यमतिवर्तते।। (च.सू. ९/२१)

- The physician should have the knowledge of Ayurveda.
- He must have a critical approach, analytical mind.
- Should have insightful understanding and special knowledge.
- Should have good memory and dedication to cure the disease.
- He should have all the practical knowledge and be able to apply it in day to day situations.

- ***Bhishaka Lakshana:***

  चिकित्सिते त्रयः पादा यस्माद्वैद्यव्यपाश्रयः।
  तस्मात् प्रयत्नमातिष्ठेद्भिषक् स्वगुणसम्पदि।। (च.सू. ९/२५)

- Medicines, nursing and patients are all dependent on the physician. So for the smooth working of the treatment process, physician should have the most sound knowledge and practical approach.

- ***Chaturvidha Vaidya Vrutti:***

मैत्री कारुण्यमार्तेषु शक्ये प्रीतिरुपेक्षणम्।
प्रकृतिस्थेषु भूतेषु वैद्यवृत्तिश्चतुर्विधेति।। (च.सू. ९/२६)

- Friendliness, sympathetic and kind towards patient, should concentrate on the diseases that can only be cured and neglect the incurable diseases.

- ***Relation of patient and doctor:***

स्त्रीभिः सहास्यां संवासं परिहासं च वर्जयेत्।
दत्तं च ताभ्यो नादेयमन्नादन्यद्भिषग्वरैः।। (सु.सू. १०/७)

- The physician should avoid sitting together with women, residing with them, making jokes with them, accept anything given by them except food.

- **Vaidya Prakar:**

1. कुवैद्योः

स्नेहादिष्वनभिज्ञो यश्छेद्यादिषु च कर्मसु।
स निहन्ति जनं लोभात् कुवैद्यो नृपदोषतः।। (सु.सू. ३/५२)

- He who is not well versed with the therapeutic procedure like oleation, surgical techniques.
- Who kills people by his greed. Such physician are known as Quacks.

2. तस्कर वैद्यः

शास्त्रं गुरुमुखोद्गीर्णमादायोपास्य चासकृत्।
यः कर्म कुरुते वैद्यः स वैद्योऽन्ये तु तस्कराः।। (सु.सू. ४/८)

- He who practices medicine after learning the science from a preceptor and engaged constantly in recapitulating it, only such is called a physician.
- While other than this qualities may show an imposter.

3. अयोग्य वैद्यः

यस्तु केवलशास्त्रज्ञः कर्मस्वपरिनिष्ठितः।
स मुह्यत्यातुरं प्राप्य प्राप्य भीरुरिवाहवम्।।
यस्तु कर्मसु निष्णातो धाष्ट्र्याच्छास्त्रबहिष्कृतः।
स सत्सु पूजां नाप्नोति वधं चर्च्छति राजतः।।
उभावेतावनिपुणावसमर्थौ स्वकर्मणि।
अर्धवेदधरावेतावेकपक्षाविव द्विजौ।।
ओषध्योऽमृतकल्पास्तु शस्त्राशनिविषोपमाः।
भवन्त्यज्ञैरुपहृतास्तस्मादेतान् विवर्जयेत्।। (सु.सू. ३/४८–५१)

- The physician who only has theoretical knowledge but lacks the practical knowledge, becomes unable to take the correct decision regarding line of treatment.
- He becomes just like a coward troop in a battle.
- He who acts opposite from the dictates of the wise, is not respected.
- These people are unable to treat the patient correctly due to their half knowledge just like a bird unable to fly having only one wing.

4. राजा योग्य वैद्यः

हेतौ लिङ्गे प्रशमने रोगाणामपुनर्भवे।
ज्ञानं चतुर्विधं यस्य स राजार्हो भिषक्तमः।। (च.सू. ६/१६)

- The physician who knows causative factor for the disease, characteristic features of disease, curative treatment for the disease and methods to prevent the reoccurrence of the disease is the best Bhishaka.
- Such a physician is said to be fit for becoming a Raja Vaidya.

5. प्राणाभिसार वैद्यः

तस्माच्छास्त्रेऽर्थविज्ञाने प्रवृत्तौ कर्मदर्शन।
भिषक् चतुष्टये युक्तः प्राणाभिसर उच्यते।। (च.सू. ६/१८)

- The physician who is engaged in the study of science, who has understood the practical aspects, who knows right methods to perform treatment, who is self-initiated in giving treatment and having abundant practical experience.
- Such a physician is known as Pranabhisara Vaidya.

6. रोगाभिसार वैद्यः

अतो विपरीता रोगाणामभिसरा हन्तारः प्राणानां,
भिषक्छद्मप्रतिच्छन्नाः कण्टकभूता लोकस्य प्रतिरूपकसधर्माणो
राज्ञां प्रमादाच्चरन्ति राष्ट्राणि।। (च.सू. २६/८)

- These physician worsen the disease and kills the person.
- They increase the Roga and decrease the life of the patient.
- These prevail in the world and injure people like thorns due to their negligence of knowledge.

- **Trividha Vaidya:**

  त्रिविधा भिषज इति– भिषक्छद्मचराः सन्ति सन्त्येके सिद्धसाधिताः।
  सन्ति वैद्यगुणैर्युक्तास्त्रिविधा भिषजो भुवि।। (च.सू. ११/५०)

- There are three types of Vaidya: Chadmachara, Siddhisadita, Vaidya Guna Yukta.
- Chadmachara and Siddhisadita are known as quacks.

***1. Chadmachara Vaidya:***

वैद्यभाण्डौषधैः पुस्तैः पल्लवैरवलोकनैः।
लभन्ते ये भिषक्शब्दमज्ञास्ते प्रतिरूपकाः।। (च.सू. ११/५१)

- These show themselves as physicians by showing the doctor's bag, a few medical books, fresh medicinal leaves.
- Though these persons are devoid of knowledge, due to their fake actions people may consider them as physicians.

***2. Siddhisadita Vaidya:***

श्रीयशोज्ञानसिद्धानां व्यपदेशादतद्विधाः।
वैद्यशब्दं लभन्ते ये ज्ञेयास्ते सिद्धसाधिताः।। (च.सू. ११/५२)

- These physicians are ignorant.
- But they get famous by boasting about their relation with the physicians who are wealthy and knowledgeable.

***3. Vaidya Guna Yukta:***

प्रयोगज्ञानविज्ञानसिद्धिसिद्धाः सुखप्रदाः।
जीविताभिसरास्ते स्युर्वैद्यत्वं तेष्ववस्थितमिति।। (च.सू. ११/५३)

- These are also called as Jivitabhisara Vaidya.
- They have all the theoretical as well as practical knowledge.
- They are well versed in giving therapeutic treatment and use their Yukti to treat the patient.
- They have infallible success and bring happiness to the life of patients by making them healthy.

- **Vaidya Sadvritta (Practice regarding social relations):**

ब्रह्मचर्यज्ञानदानमैत्रीकारुण्यहर्षोपेक्षाप्रशमपरश्च स्यादिति।।
(च.सू. ८/२९)

- One should follow celibacy, knowledge, donation, compassion, empathy, happiness, detachment and peace.

Table 16.1

| | |
|---|---|
| न कार्यकालमतिपातयेत् | Should not postpone things at the time of action |
| नापरीक्षितमभिनिविशेत् | Never take up anything without examining it |
| नेन्द्रियवशगः स्यात् | Not be submissive to his sense organs |
| न चञ्चलं मनोऽनुभ्रामयेत्, | Not be trickle minded |
| बुद्धीन्द्रियाणामतिभारमादध्यात् | Never over-burden the sense organs |
| न चातिदीर्घसूत्री स्यात्, | Not be too much dilatory |
| न क्रोधहर्षावनुविदध्यात् | Not act under anger or exhilaration |
| न शोकमनुवसेत् | Not live under a continuous grief |
| न सिद्धावुत्सेकं,<br>यच्छेन्नासिद्धौ दैन्य | Not be exhilarated in success or depressed in failure |
| प्रकृतिमभीक्ष्णं स्मरेत्, | Always keep constitutional in mind |

| | |
|---|---|
| हेतुप्रभावनिश्चितः स्याद्धेत्वारम्भनित्यश्च | Be confident of the effect of cause and initiate the cause |
| न कृतमित्याश्वसेत् | Never assume that nothing can work now |
| न वीर्यं जह्यात् | Never give up the courage |
| नापवादमनुस्मरेत् | Never remember the blame |

- ***Ethics of medical practice:***
    - The laws regarding medical practice vary from country to country.
    - The board principles of medical ethics are universal and are formulated by World Medical Association (WMA).

***International code of medical ethics for doctors:***
- World Medical Association, Geneva 1893 stated "A physician should preserve confidentiality on all he knows about his patients even after the patient has died.
- In India, the registered medical practitioner should always follow the regulations of council.
- This also gives the direction to not disclose the secrets of patients that have been learnt in the exercise of his profession except in a court of law or in notifiable diseases.

***1. Charak oath:***
- Young doctors take the Charak oath before starting their medical practice.

अथैनमग्निसकाशे ब्राह्मणसकाशे भिषक्सकाशे चानुशिष्यात्:

- Teacher should instruct the disciple in the presence of sacred fire, brahmanas and physicians.

ब्रह्मचारिणा श्मश्रुधारिण सत्यवादिनाऽमांसादेन मेध्यसेविना
निर्मत्सरेणाशस्त्रधारिणा च भवितव्यं, न च ते मद्वचनात् किञ्चिदकार्यं

स्यादन्यत्र राजद्विष्टात् प्राणहराद्विपुलादधर्म्यादनर्थसम्प्रयुक्ताद्वाऽप्यर्थात्ः

- Should lead the life of a bachelor, should grow hair and beard, speak only the truth, should not have meat intake, should eat food only made of pure articles, should not envy about others, not carry any arms.
- Should not do any act of great unrighteousness or leads to calamity.

मदर्पणेन मत्प्रधानेन मदधीनेन मत्प्रियहितानुवर्तिना च शश्वद्भवितव्यं, पुत्रवद्दासवदर्थिवच्चोपचरताऽनुवस्तव्योऽहम्,अनुत्सेकेनावहितेनानन्यमनसा विनीतेनावेक्ष्यावेक्ष्यकारिणाऽनसूयकेन चाभ्यनुज्ञातेन प्रविचरितव्यम्, अनुज्ञातेन (चाननुज्ञातेन च) प्रविचरता पूर्वं गुर्वर्थोपाहरणे यथाशक्ति प्रयतितव्यं;

- One should behave without arrogance and be respectful, be careful and attentive.
- With undistracted mind, humility, constant reflection and with ungrudging obedience.
- Should be at their best behavior and conduct all the activities to achieve the goal of their teacher's purpose with their best ability.

कर्मसिद्धिमर्थसिद्धं यशोलाभं प्रेत्य च स्वर्गमिच्छता भिषजा त्वया गोब्राह्मणमादौ कृत्वा सर्वप्राणभृतां शर्माशासितव्यमहरहरुत्तिष्ठता चोपविशता च,

- If one desires success, wealth, fame as physicians and heaven after the death, then they should pray for the welfare of all the creatures starting from cows and brahmanas.

सर्वात्मना चातुराणामारोग्याय प्रयतितव्यं, जीवितहेतोरपि चातुरेभ्यो नाभिद्रोग्धव्यं, मनसाऽपि च परस्त्रियो नाभिगमनीयास्तथा सर्वमेव परस्वं, निभृतवेशपरिच्छदेन भवितव्यम्, अशौण्डेनापापेनापापसहायेन च, श्लक्ष्णशुक्लध

र्यशर्म्यधन्यसत्यहितमितवचसा देशकालविचारिणा स्मृतिमता ज्ञानोत्थानोपकरण ासम्पत्सु नित्यं यत्नवता च;

- Day and night they should be engaged to treat patients with all their heart and soul.
- Should never injure patients for the sake of one's life or living.
- Should never commit adultery.
- Be modest in there attire and appearance.
- Should never be drunk, never have the company of a sinful man or any criminals.
- Should always speak truth, use humble and pleasing words.
- Their behaviour must be according to time and place. Be heedful of the past experiences.

न च कदाचिद्राजद्विष्टानां राजद्वेषिणां वा महाजनद्विष्टानां महाजनद्वेषिणां वाऽप्यौषधमनुविधातव्यं, तथा
सर्वेषामत्यर्थविकृतदुष्टदुःखशीलाचारोपचाराणामनपवादप्रतिकारणां (२) मुमूर्षूणां च, तथैवासन्निहितेश्वराणां स्त्रीणामनध्यक्षाणां वा;

- No person who is hated by the king, or has hate towards king or is hated by the public shall receive treatment.
- Those with a miserable or wicked character, who are disrespectful, who are on the verge of death, women who are unaccompanied by their husband or guardians shall not receive the treatment.

न च कदाचित् स्त्रीदत्तमामिषमादातव्यमननुज्ञातं भर्त्राऽथवाऽध्यक्षेण, आतुरकुलं चानुप्रविशता विदितेनानुमतप्रवेशिना सार्धं पुरुषेण सुसंवीतेनावाक्शिरसा स्मृतिमता स्तिमितेनावेक्ष्यावेक्ष्य मनसा सर्वमाचरता सम्यगनुप्रवेष्टव्यम्, अनुप्रविश्य च वाङ्मनोबुद्धीन्द्रियाणि न क्वचित् प्रणिधातव्यान्यन्यत्रातुरादातुरोपकारार्थादातुरगतेष्वन्येषु वा भावेषु, न चातुरकुलप्रवृत्तयो बहिर्निश्चारयितव्याः, ह्रसितं चायुषः प्रमाणमातुरस्य जानताऽपि त्वया न वर्णयितव्यं तत्र यत्रोच्यमानमातुरस्यान्यस्य वाऽप्युपघाताय सम्पद्यते;

- Not to offer the meat offered by a woman not accompanied by her husband.
- While entering the patient's house, one should be accompanied by a known person who has the permission to enter the patient's house.
- After entering the patient's house mind, actions, thoughts be only of helping the patient out of his miserable disease.
- The physician should not mention anything serious about the health on the spot.

ज्ञानवताऽपि च नात्यर्थमात्मनो ज्ञाने विकत्थितव्यम्, आप्तादपि हि विकत्थमानादत्यर्थमुद्विजन्त्यनेके.

- Never boast about the knowledge one has.
- Even the good and authoritative persons are offended by boasting too much about the knowledge.

न चैव ह्यस्ति सुतरमायुर्वेदस्य पारं, तस्मादप्रमत्तः शश्वदभियोगमस्मिन् गच्छेत्, एतच्च कार्यम्, एवम्भूयश्च वृत्तसौष्ठवमनसूयता परेभ्योऽप्यागमयितव्यं, कृत्स्नो हि लोको बुद्धिमतामाचार्यः शत्रुश्चाबुद्धिमताम्, अतश्चाभिसमीक्ष्य बुद्धिमताऽमित्रस्यापि धन्यं यशस्यमायुष्यं पौष्टिकं लौक्यमभ्युपदिशतो वचः श्रोतव्यमनुविधातव्यं चेति.

- There is no limitation to the science of life. So one should apply it diligently.
- The entire world is a teacher to the intelligent and a foe for people not interested in knowledge.
- Thus one must learn good things even from the enemy, when they are worthy and gives fame and long life.

अतः परमिदं ब्रूयात्– देवताग्निद्विजगुरुवृद्धसिद्धाचार्येषु ते नित्यं सम्यग्वर्तितव्यं, तेषु ते सम्यग्वर्तमानस्यायमग्निः सर्वगन्धरसरत्नबीजानि यथेरिताश्च देवताः शिवाय स्युः, अतोऽन्यथा वर्तमानस्याशिवायेति.

- One should be respectful towards God, teachers, sacred fire, twice born, aged.

- If the person becomes disrespectful, then remains abstained from knowledge, success and fame.

एवं ब्रुवति चाचार्ये शिष्यः 'तथा' इति ब्रूयात्.
यथोपदेशं च कुर्वन्नध्याप्यः, अतोऽन्यथा त्वनध्याप्यः.
अध्याप्यमध्यापयन् ह्याचार्यो यथोक्तैश्चाध्यापनफलैर्योगमाप्नोत्यन्यैश्चानुक्तैः
श्रेयस्करैर्गुणैः शिष्यमात्मानं च युनक्ति. इत्यध्यापनविधिरुक्तः ।

- The student must agree to the teacher's above given instructions.
- He who follows the instructions is only to be taught while others are not.
- The teacher who teaches a worthy and an obedient disciple obtains all the auspicious results of teaching.

***2. Hippocratic oath:***

- "I swear by Apollo the physician, and Aesculapius the surgeon, likewise Hygeia and Panacea, and call all the gods and goddesses to witness, that I will observe and keep this underwritten oath, to the utmost of my power and judgment.
- I will reverence my master who taught me the art. Equally with my parents, will I allow him things necessary for his support, and will consider his sons as brothers. I will teach them my art without reward or agreement; and I will impart all my acquirement, instructions, and whatever I know, to my master's children, as to my own; and likewise to all my pupils, who shall bind and tie themselves by a professional oath, but to none else.
- With regard to healing the sick, I will devise and order for them the best diet, according to my judgment and means; and I will take care that they suffer no hurt or damage. Nor shall any man's entreaty prevail upon me to administer poison to anyone; neither will I counsel any man to do so. Moreover, I will give no sort of medicine to any pregnant woman, with a

view to destroy the child. Further, I will comport myself and use my knowledge in a godly manner.

- I will not cut for the stone, but will commit that affair entirely to the surgeons.
- Whatsoever house I may enter, my visit shall be for the convenience and advantage of the patient; and I will willingly refrain from doing any injury or wrong from falsehood, and (in an especial manner) from acts of an amorous nature, whatever may be the rank of those who it may be my duty to cure, whether mistress or servant, bond or free.
- Whatever, in the course of my practice, I may see or hear (even when not invited), whatever I may happen to obtain knowledge of, if it be not proper to repeat it, I will keep sacred and secret within my own breast. If I faithfully observe this oath, may I thrive and prosper in my fortune and profession, and live in the estimation of posterity; or on breach thereof, may the reverse be my fate!"

## *16.2 NCISM: Constitution, objectives and functions:*

- **Constitution of NCISM:**
  - In the persuade of provisions of National Commission for Indian System of Medicine Act 2020, the Indian Medicine Central Council Act 1970, has been repealed and all the previous provisions of NCISM has been come into force from the 11$^{th}$ day of June, 2021.
  - Under the previous section of 59 (2) of NCISM Act 2020, the central government has constituted the commission and 4 other autonomous board on the same day.
  - Medical standards and other requirements of IMCC 1970 and the rules & regulations made there under shall continue to be in force and will continue till new standards or requirements as specified under the new act made, come into force.

- However, the provisions of the following regulations which are in-consistent with the provisions of NCISM Act 2020 shall not be applicable.

- **Objectives of NCISM:**
    - Improve the access of quality and affordable Ayurveda, Unani, Siddha, Sowa-Rigpa medical education.
    - Ensure availability of adequate and high quality of AUS&SR medical professionals in all part of country.
    - Promote equitable and universal health care that encourages community health perspectives.
    - Allow medical professionals to update to latest medical research in their work and contribute to research.
    - Objectively rate and access medical institutions regularly in a transparent manner.
    - Maintain a national AUS&SR register for India.
    - Enforce high ethical standards in all aspects of AUS&SR medical services.
    - Have an effective grievance redressed mechanism.

- **Functions of NCISM:**
    - To provide medical education system that improves access to quality and affordable medical education.
    - To ensure the availability of adequate and high quality of medical professionals in Indian System of Medicine.
    - To promote national health goals.
    - Promote equitable and universal health care that encourages community health perspectives.
    - Allow medical professionals to update to latest medical research in their work and contribute to research.
    - To carry out periodic and transparent assessment of medical institutions.
    - To provide medical education system that is flexible to the changing needs and has effective redressed

mechanism.

### 16.3 Duties, rights and privileges of a Registered Medical Practitioner:

- ***Duties of RMP:***
    - Respect a competent patient's right to accept or refuse a treatment.
    - Deal honestly with patients and colleagues.
    - Not receive any financial benefits for referring patients or prescribing a specific product.
    - Behave towards colleagues as one wants to have others behave towards them.
    - Provide a high quality practice and care at all times.

- ***Rights and privileges of RMP:***
    - To practice medicine.
    - To choose patient.
    - To prescribe or dispense medicines.
    - To possess, prescribe or dispense drugs enlisted in the Dangerous Drug Act.
    - To add professional titles to his name.
    - To perform surgical operations, to prescribe certificate.
    - To give evidence as an expert witness in the court of law.
    - To claim fees for the professional services given.

- ***Rights and privileges of patients:***
    - To choose doctor.
    - To access the health care facilities regardless of age, sex, caste, religion.
    - To be treated with dignity, care, respect and without discrimination.
    - To have privacy during consultation or treatment.
    - To receive complete information about diagnosis,

investigations and best methods of treatment.
  - To have confidentiality of all his informations given to doctor.
  - To know the procedure of operation, risk involved, suitable alternatives, type of procedure, safety of procedure, results and prognosis.
  - To seek second opinion from another doctor.
  - To demand for medical record.
  - To complain and have rectification of grievances.
  - To receive compensation for medical injuries or negligence.

### 16.4 Consent, professional secrecy and privileged communication:

- ***Consent:***
  - A free and voluntary agreement or permission given for a special act or purpose.
  - Consent is based on trust, openness and good communication.
  - It is a key concept of healthcare.
  - All the decisions of investigation or treatment should come as a result of collaboration between doctor and patient.
  - If the patient is unable to make the decision, the person close to the patient gives consent.

- ***Importance of consent:***
  - The patient has the right to give or not the permission of examination, investigation, treatment, surgery or research.
  - It is highly necessary before treating a patient or performing surgery.
  - Without the consent, examination or treatment is considered as an assault as all the people have right to

decide what shall be done to his body by rule of self defence of body (IPC 96-102, 104 provides the right to the bodily integrity of the patient by others).

- ***Professional secrecy:***
- It is the duty of doctor not to share any information about his patients except for the situations below:

1. In a court of law, under the orders of presiding judge.
2. Privileged communication.
3. Notifiable diseases.

- ***Privileged communication:***
    - A communication between doctor and patient which is protected from public disclosure.
    - The conversation be disclosed if doctor is concerned about criminal acts being committed against others which could be prevented by the disclosure to proper authorities.

## 16.5 Professional negligence, professional misconduct, unethical practices:

- ***Medical negligence:***
    - It is the failure to execute reasonable degree of skill and care or a wilfully negligence by medical practitioner which causes harm, bodily injury or death of patient.

Table 16.2 Acts of negligence

| Act of commission | Act of omission |
|---|---|
| Doing something a reasonable and responsible practitioner would never do. | Not doing something that a reasonable and responsible practitioner would do in a given circumstance. |

**1. Doctrine of Res Ipsa Loquitur:**

- This means that the thing speaks for itself.
- Here the patient need not prove anything as the doctor would be directly held guilty.
- This is applied according to the doctrine of common know.
- Can be applied in both civil and criminal suits.
- Eg: Operation of a wrong patient or a wrong part, forgotten instruments, mismatch transfusion, loss of hand due to prolong splinting.

**2. Novus Actus Intervenens:**

- This means unrelated act intervening.
- There is always a logical sequence of treatment. If the continuity broken due to negligence, it leads to unexpected circumstances.
- Eg: Patient goes to a doctor and gets prescribed medicine. The same patient visits another doctor and intakes drugs given by him causing a reaction.
- In this case, the first doctor won't be held guilty.

Table 16.3 Types of medical negligence

| **Civil negligence** | **Criminal negligence** |
|---|---|
| No specific law violation. | Clear violence of law. |
| Simple absence of skill and care. | Gross absence of skill and care. |
| Consent : good defence. | Consent : not a defence. |
| Civil court trial. | Criminal court trial. |
| Strong evidence is sufficient. | Guilt should be proven. |
| Punishment be to pay the damage. | Punishment be 2 years imprisonment. |

- **Defences against medical negligence:**

***1. Calculated risk doctrine:***

- An element of risk is there in all surgeries.
- Injury may occur even though reasonable skill is present and

care is taken.
- Eg: 5-10% deaths occur in pulmonary transplant surgeries.

***2. Contributory negligence:***
- An unreasonable conduct on the part of patient along with the negligence of doctor causing injury.
- Eg: Patient does not give history of drug allergy.

***3. Corporate negligence:***
- The hospital management fails to provide adequate facility.
- Not providing standard equipment and skilled employees.
- The hospital has to pay the damage.

***4. Medical mal-occurrence:***
- Inevitable accidents occur even if adequate care, precautions and skilful doctor present.
- Eg: Amniotic fluid embolism during LSCS.

***Professional misconduct:***
- Adultery or misconduct when done with the patient, the physician of Indian medicine is liable for disciplinary action against him.
- If convicted for selling scheduled poison to anyone under his own qualification except his patients is liable for disciplinary actions.
- Performing illegal abortion or illegal operation for which there is no medical, surgical or psychological indication.
- Should not have an unusually large sign board or writing anything except his name, university of qualification, title and name of his speciality. The same should be followed on his prescription papers.
- Do not disclose the secrets of patients that has been learnt in the exercise of the profession. It can be disclosed only under the court of law on orders of presiding judge.

- Refusing on the religion backgrounds alone to give assistance in sterility, birth controls, craniotomy in living children, therapeutic abortion under the medical indication.
- Before conducting any procedure the consent should be obtained in writing by parents or guardians in case of minor. The surgery which may cause sterility the consent of wife and husband is needed compulsory.
- The case reports or details of any patient should not be published in any journal which can reveal the identity of patient.
- Shall not exhibit the fee scale publicly. But same can be displayed in waiting or consulting rooms.
- Advertisements and tour programs are both unethical.

***Unethical practices:***

- No medical practice in law is allowed without registered license.
- Irrational prescriptions: should be conversant with the side effects and complications of medicines.
- No drugs which have expired the manufacturer's specifications be dispensed to the patients.
- Practicing a procedure beyond the formal training.
- The laws of Malawi refuses to terminate the pregnancy.
- Before any procedure the consent be taken. But before a major procedure, an informed written consent be taken.
- Negligence in diagnosis or treatment: failing to visit a patient without making an alternate arrangement.
- Stigmatization and discrimination: based on religion, race, sex, age and people living with HIV.
- Theft of medical supplies.
- Ethical dilemmas: Patient's refusal of treatment, withdrawal of active treatment, confidentiality, patient or pain killing.

## 16.6 Defences in medical negligence suits:

- As per section 375 of CrPC, there is provision of compensation along with imprisonment or other penalty as described by IPC.
- But in August 2005, the Supreme Court of India gave a judgement, "**no doctor can be arrested on simply filling the complaint against him by any patient or relative of the patient. His arrest can only be there if needed for furthering the investigation or for collecting evidence or investigating officer thinks that doctor may run away to evade arrest.**"
- The judgement also gives the direction for the preceding officer before proceeding against the doctor "**the investigating officer should obtain an independent and competent opinion preferably from a doctor in government service qualified in that branch of medical practice.**"

## 16.7 Medical records:

- The legal document providing a chronicles of patient's medical history and care.
- Physician, nurse practitioner, nurses and other members of health care teams may make entries in the records.

***Components of medical records:***

- Identification summary sheet.
- Consent for treatments.
- Legal documents: referral letter, request for information.
- Discharge summary, referral slip.
- Admission notes, clinical progress note, operation report if operation has been performed.
- Investigation reports like X-ray, pathology, etc.
- Orders for treatment and medication forms listing daily medications ordered and given with the signature of doctor prescribing the medicines.

***Uses of medical records:***

Table 16.4

| Requirement for doctor | Requirement for patient |
|---|---|
| Follow up cases. | Follow up cases or treatment from another doctor. |
| Planning for further treatment. | Medico legal cases or medical negligence cases. |
| Evaluation of drug therapy. | For life insurance policy cases. |
| For medical research. | As a proof of disability. |
| Hospital audit, administration, health insurance. | For third party claims. |

***Preparation of medical records:***

- A report may be requested by the police prosecutor, coroners, judges, medical administrators, government departments, city authorities or lawyers.
- Whenever the medical records may be required to review, written permission to access and use those records has been given either by individual themselves or body with that power to give consent.
- The fact of request even from court not mean that a doctor can necessarily ignore the rules of medical confidentiality.
- Mandatory reporting of medical issues may be relevant in some countries often related to child abuse, violent crimes.

***Structure of statement:***

- The basis of most reports and statements lies in the notes made simultaneously.
- A simple professional witness statement may include doctor's professional address and qualification may follow.
- The date of report is essential. Time(s), date(s), place(s) of examination(s) be listed as should the details of any other person present while examination.

- Medical abbreviation should be used with care and highly technical terms those related to complex pieces of equipment be explained in simple terms.
- Autopsy reports are a special type of reports and may be occasional by the coroner, police or legally competent person. It is confidential report which may only be disclosed to the examining authority.
- Doctors must resist any attempt to change or delete any part of their report by lawyers, any request to re-write or re-submit a report with alterations be refused.

## 16.8 Consumer Protection Act:

- The Consumer Protection Act 1986 was introduced with the purpose to provide relief to the consumer against erring traders and manufacturers
- There was a need for consumers be protected against wrong business practices.
- The act intends to provide cheap and speedy trials for consumer benefits, as it was found that civil courts were already burdened with heavy work.
- The law defines obligations of manufacturers and traders.
- Any Consumer who feels that service is not provided to him for which he has paid is entitled for relief.

### *1. District forum:*

- Has three members: The chairman either a siting district or session judge, other two members are eminent citizens one being a lady.
- Can award a compensation upto Rs.20 lakhs.

### *2. State level forum:*

- Known as State Consumer Redressal Commission.
- It is presided by a sitting High court judge or retired one.
- Other two are eminent citizens, one being a lady member.

- Appeal against the district consumer forum are heard here.
- Can award a compensation upto Rs. 1 Crore.

***3. National level forum:***

- National Consumer Redressal Commission is in New Delhi.
- It is precided by a sitting Supreme Court judge or a retired one.
- Other members are eminent citizens, one being a lady member.
- The commission can award any amount of compensation.
- Appeal against the National Consumer Redressal Commission are heard in Supreme Court.

***Procedure to file complaint:***

- The procedure to file a complaint is very simple. There is no need of any lawyer.
- No Court fee is required. Application on a plain paper is sufficient along with copy of goods purchased.
- The judgement would be given in 90 days but now there are many pending results causing delay in justice.
- The complaint has to be filed in 2 years of cause of action. But the court has the powers to admit the case even after 2 years if it finds reason of delay valid.
- The act allows provisions for establishing councils at state and central level for protection of consumers.
- The salient features of judgement are:
    1. Hospitals and doctors which render service without any charge to every person will not fall under the purview of service.
    2. If hospital is charging a token amount for registration but providing free services to everyone, it would not cover under the Act.
    3. Services rendered by doctors and hospitals or nursing homes on payment basis falls under the Act.
    4. Doctors, hospitals or nursing homes providing free

services to poor class but the bulk service is rendered onto the patient also comes under the Act.

5. When a person has taken medical insurance policy for treatment where all the charges for consultation, diagnosis and treatments are borne by the insurance company, here the person receiving treatment is beneficiary of the service which has been rendered by medical practitioner. The payment for which would be met by insurance company under the insurance policy. The service would not be free of charge and thus the given service is defined under the Act.
6. Government dispensaries where services are rendered on payment of charges and also rendered free of charges to other persons availing such services would fall under the Act.
7. Services rendered free in government hospitals, dispensaries will not be covered under the Act. Such government doctors or dispensaries would be outside the purview of consumer forum. The services however paid for like pathology, radiology or any diagnostic procedures, when fee is charged by the hospital falls under the Act.

**Multiple Choice Questions**

**1. NCISM came into force in which year?**

A. 2018 B. 2019 C. 2021 D. 2022

**2. District forum can award compensation upto how many rupees?**

A. 20 lakhs B. 50 lakhs C. 10 crore D. 25 crore

**3.** हेतौ लिङ्गे प्रशमने रोगाणामपुनर्भवे | **shows the quality of which Vaidya?**

A.अयोग्य वैद्यः B. कुवैद्यो

C. राजा योग्य वैद्यः D.प्राणाभिसार वैद्यः

**4. Appeal against the National Consumer Redressal Commission are heard in ?**

A. District court B. High court C. Supreme court D. None

**5. The hospital management fails to provide adequate facility shows which type of negligence?**

A. Contributory B. Corporate

C. Mal occurrence D. Risk doctrine

**6. These physician worsen the disease and kills the person shows which Vaidya type?**

A. रोगाभिसार वैद्यः B. कुवैद्यो C. अयोग्य वैद्यः D. प्राणाभिसार वैद्यः

**7. Which of the following does not come under Trividha Vaidya?**

A. Pranabhisara B. Chadmachara

C. Siddhisadita D. Vaidya Guna yukta

**8. Consumer Protection Act was introduced in which year?**

A. 1981 B. 1975 C. 1999 D. 1986

**9. As per which section of CrPC, there is provision of compensation along with imprisonment?**

A. 370 B. 375 C. 301 D. 308

**10. National Consumer Redressal Commission is situated at?**

A. New Delhi B. Hyderabad C. Jaipur D. Lucknow

**Answer key for MCQs:**

| | |
|---|---|
| 1 | C |
| 2 | A |
| 3 | C |
| 4 | C |
| 5 | B |

| | |
|---|---|
| 6 | A |
| 7 | A |
| 8 | D |
| 9 | B |
| 10 | A |

# Ch. 17
# Legal Procedures

## 17.1 Courts and their powers:

- ***Courts in India:***
    - India has one of the efficient Judiciary systems.
    - The existence of court is required to check the misuse of powers.
    - Court includes and signifies the person, legally authorized to record evidence and give a judgement.

Image 17.1

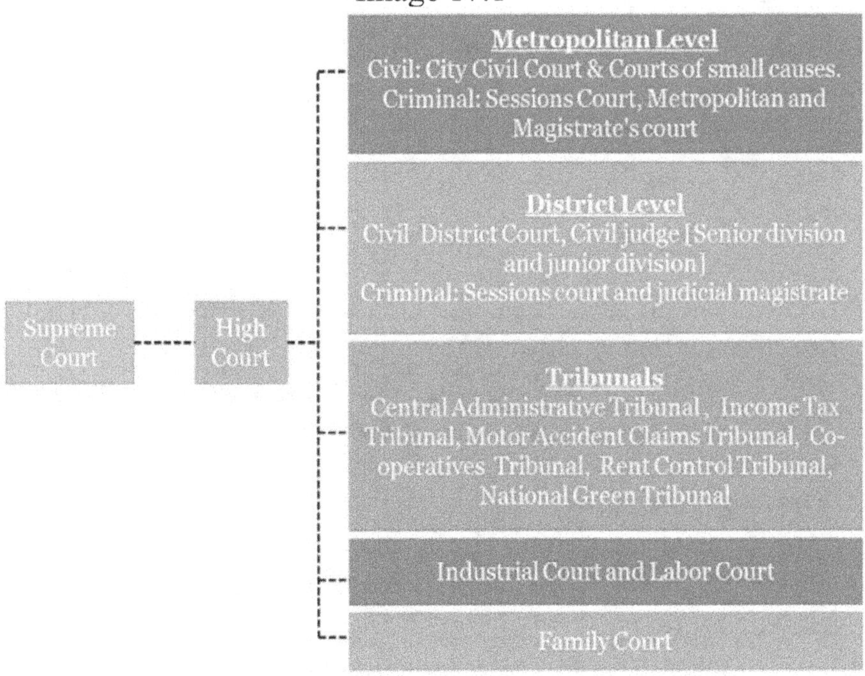

Image 17.2

**Hierarchy of Judges in India.**

Chief Justice of India

(Supreme Court)

↓

Chief Justice of High Courts

↓

District Judge/ Sessions Judge

↓ ↓

| Civil Court | Criminal Court |
|---|---|
| (Senior Civil Judge) | (Chief Judicial Magistrate/ Metropolitan Judge) |
| ↓ | ↓ |
| Principal Junior Civil Judge | Judicial Magistrate II Class/ Metropolitan Magistrate I class |
| ↓ | |
| Junior Civil Judge/Munsif Court | |

***Criminal court:***

- Deals with the disputes between the State and individual as per IPC.
- It deals with the offenses which are considered against the public interest.
- Eg: Kidnapping, robbery, rape, criminal abortion.
- There are 4 types of criminal courts in India:

***1. The Supreme court:***

- Highest judicial tribunal in India.
- It can pass any sentence and usually considers appeals from lower courts.
- It can sustain or alter the punishment approved by the high court.

***2. The High court:***

- Highest judicial tribunal in the state and usually located in capital of the state.
- It can pass any sentence prescribed by law.
- Any jurisdiction given by sessions court can be appealed here

***3. The Sessions court:***

- Located in district headquarters and can pass any sentence authorized by law.
- Additional sessions judge and assistant sessions judge appointed by high court passes the sentence in this court.

***4. The Magistrate court:***

*A. Chief Judicial Magistrate:*

- This is first class officer appointed by high court in metropolitan area.
- It can pass any sentence excluding imprisonment to death, lifetime imprisonment or imprisonment more than 7 years.
- Can pass sentence with any amount of fine.

*B. First Class Judicial Magistrate:*

- This could pass the sentence of imprisonment for a term not exceeding 3 years or a fine not exceeding 10,000 or both

*C. Second Class Judicial Magistrate:*

- State government may establish after permission of high court.
- This could pass a sentence of imprisonment for a term not exceeding 1 year or fine not exceeding 5000 or both.

*D. Juvenile court:*

- These are the special courts which try offenses committed by juvenile (below 18 years of age).

***Civil court:***

- Deals with the disputes between individual including those of alleged negligence, debt, land disputes, divorce, education.
- Decisions made by judges are referred to as common law.
- In both civil and criminal trials, the person against whom the action is being taken is called the defendant.

***Consumer court:***

- It deals with the consumer disputes with powers similar to civil court.

Table 17.1

| **Consumer court** | **Fine limit** |
|---|---|
| District forum | Less than 20 lakhs |
| State commission | 20 lakhs – 1 crore |
| National commission | More than 1 crore |

***Coroner's court:***

- It was only present at Mumbai and Kolkata which only dealt with inquest.
- Now it is abolished at both the places, having no coroner's court in India.

## 17.2 Inquest, evidences, eye witnesses, offenses

***Inquest :***

- A judicial inquiry to ascertain the facts relaying to an incidence or an investigation into something that has happened.
- It is conducted by Judge, jury or government official. Autopsy may be required to be carried out by medical examiner.

Table 17.2 Types of inquest

| **Police inquest** | **Magistrate inquest** | **Medical examiner's system** |
|---|---|---|
| -Under Section 174 CrPC. | • Under Section 176 CrPC. | • Done in the USA and not in India. |
| -Police officer is the investigating officer who collects information from public, informers. | • Carried out by executive or district magistrate. | • A medical person is appointed to do the inquest. |
| -After informing the nearest executive magistrate, he goes to site of crime to conduct inquest. | • This type of inquest is considered superior to the police inquest. | • He visits the scene if crime and collects of the first hand evidences and interprets them by applying the medical knowledge. |
| -In presence of 2 or more Pancha, prepare Panchanama. | • Carried in conditions like: | • To find out the result, autopsy may be considered. |
| -Panchanama.is signed by police officer and witnesses. | • Death in prison, reformatories, brostal schools. | • Better than other inquest where non medical person conducts it. |
| -If no suspect found, body given to relatives. If suspect found sent for PM examination.<br>Eg: Murder, accident, homicidal poisoning. | • Death due to police firing, death under police custody during interrogation. | • He submits his report to the district attorney. |
| -Investigating officer summons the person who must attend to give answer to the inquiry. | • Dowry death: less than 30 years of age and within 7 years of marriage. | |
| -Otherwise he may be punished under IPC section 179. | • Death in psychiatric hospital, person disappears or alleged rape.<br>• If the government wants for any case. | |

***Evidence :***

- It can be a statement or report.
- A statement in a criminal case is a report that is prepared in a particular form so that it can be used as evidence.
- A statement may be accepted by both defence and prosecution, negating the need for court attendance.

***Medical evidence:***

- A written document or oral report by a medical science which helps the court to decide a case.

A. Written: medical certificate, dying declaration, dying deposition, medico-legal reports.

B. Oral: direct and indirect.

C. Circumstantial

Table 17.3

| **Medical certificate** | **Medico-legal reports** | **Dying declaration** | **Dying deposition** |
|---|---|---|---|
| -Issued by medical officer at request of patient or his relatives. | -Prepared by RMP at request of investigating officer or court. | -In presence of executive officer, doctor, village head.<br>--It is recorded in presence of 2 uninterested witness. | -It is the statement recorded by magistrate of a person on oath in presence of accused. |
| -For birth, sickness, fitness purpose. | -It is considered as evidence when doctor testify under oath.<br>Eg: Report of age, injury, impotence. | -If a person recorded his statement written or oral who is likely to die unnaturally saying circumstances. | -His lawyer is allowed to cross examine the witness.<br>-Retains full value even when person does not die. |

***Oral evidence:***

- When evidence given orally under the oath in a court of law.
- This is superior to written evidence because in court cross examination is possible.

***Circumstantial evidence:***

- When an evidence is collected from circumstances or surrounding of a case.
- Eg: suicidal note, finger print  foot print, bullet.

***Witness:***

- A person who gives sworn testimony or evidence in the court of law for any fact under inquiry.
- A person who gives evidence under the oath in a court of law is called witness.
- However the expert witness be impartial and unbiased in his assessment.

Table 17.4

| **Common witness** | **Expert witness** |
|---|---|
| • One who gives evidence to the facts observed, heard or perceived by him. | • A person who by his professional training is capable of forming opinions. |
| | • Draws a conclusion from the facts observed.<br>Eg; Handwriting expert, ballistic expert, chemical analyzer.[7] |

**Offenses:**

Table 17.5 Types of offenses

| Cognizable offense | Non cognizable offense |
|---|---|
| -Police can arrest a person without a warrant. | -Warrant from a magistrate is necessary for arrest of a person. |
| Eg: rape, murder, dowry death. | Eg: defamation, minor assault, public nuisance |

## 17.3 Court procedure: summons, oath, recording of evidence and conduct money:

***Summons:***

- A legal document compelling attendance of witness in a court of law under penalty in a fixed day and place for giving evidence.
- Issued by the court in writing, in duplicate, signed and sealed by preceding officer of the court

***Oath:***

- Declaration required by law and is compulsory to take by every witness respon for evidence given.
- By putting hands on religious books Geetaji (Hindu), Quran (Muslim), Bible (Christian).
- Saying " I swear by God that I shall speak truth, the whole truth and nothing else but the truth.
- If the witness is found false is called as perjury, the person is punishable with crime under Section 193 IPC and imprisonment for upto 7 years and fine.
- A child below 12 years is not required to take oath.

***Recording of evidence:***

a. Examination in chief: Witness will be the first to examine under oath.
b. Cross examination: When thus questioning is completed, the other lawyers will have the opportunity to question to the

witness. This tests the evidence already given.

c. Re-examination and court's question: The final pattern of giving evidence is re-examination. The original lawyer has the opportunity to clarify anything that has been raised in cross examination.

***Conduct money:***

- Traveling expense to reach the court for the summons in civil cases is paid by the party called for evidence.

## 17.4 Conduct of a medical professional in court of law:

1. As a expert witness, to support a medical opinion already secured, to explain medical condition of a party, witness in civil or criminal cases or in actions complaining about medical negligence.
2. As accused in a criminal case for commission of offenses under one or other penal laws.
3. A medical professional having a law degree wishing to pursue practice as a lawyer.

***Duties of a doctor in witness box:***

- Well prepared with the details of evidence before entering the box.
- Take all records and relevant reports like original notes, autopsy reports, X-rays, photographs, copy of death certificate, swabs reports, smear reports.
- These should be taken notes of before entering the witness box as they may have to be quoted.

**Multiple Choice Questions**

**1. Perjury is punishable under which section of IPC?**

A. 110 B. 175 C. 193 D. 206

**2. A child below what years of age does not require to take oath in witness box?**

A. 15 B. 13 C. 17 D. 12

**3. Magistrate inquest comes under which section of CrPC?**

A. 176 B. 175 C. 173 D. 179

**4. District forum can charge fine upto what amount?**

A. 50 lakhs B. 2 crore C. 10 lakhs D. 45 crore

**5. Juvenile court comes under what classification of courts?**

A. High court B. Supreme court
C. Sessions court D. Magistrate court

**6. First class judicial magistrate cannot pass sentence of imprisonment above?**

A. 2 years B. 3 years C. 5 years D. 7 years

**7. Criminal court does not deal with?**

A. Land disputes B. Kidnapping C. Rape D. Robbery

**8. Second Class Judicial Magistrate can give fine upto what amount?**

A. 8000 B. 2000 C. 5000 D. 3000

**9. A legal document compelling attendance of witness in a court of law is?**

A. Summons B. Oath C. Penalty D. Evidence

**10. A written document or oral report by a medical science which helps the court to decide a case is?**

A. Medical evidence B. Oath

C. Summons D. Conduct money

**Answer key for MCQs:**

| 1 | C |
|---|---|
| 2 | D |
| 3 | A |
| 4 | C |
| 5 | D |

| 6 | B |
|---|---|
| 7 | A |
| 8 | C |
| 9 | B |
| 10 | A |

# Ch. 18
# Personal Identity

## 18.1 Identification Data:

Identification: Identification is the determination or establishment of the identity of a person whether living or dead.

• *Types: - 2*

**i) Complete / Absolute:** Exact determination of the identity of a person.

**ii) Incomplete / Partial:** Incomplete determination of the identity of a person.

- **Medico-legal Aspects:** Identification required in: Suspected foul play, assault, rape, disputed sex, false personification to secure property, insurance, pension and fragmented remains of body in mass fatalities.

***Identification:***

- Religion
- Race
- Sex
- Age
- Blood grouping
- Stature
- Tattoo marks
- Scars
- Teeth
- Deformities

- Anthropometry
- Foot prints
- Cheiloscopy
- Poroscopy

## 18.2 Age

*Age:*

- For the determination of age, the following data should be collected:

***Height & weight:***

These are no very reliable means of estimating the age of an individual. Comparison of the person's measurement with standard height & weight charts will

only give a rough idea of the age. In case of foetus or new-born child, height & weight are of greater importance.

- **Number of teeth:** Teeth form a reliable means of estimating the age of an individual up to 25 years because different teeth erupt at different definite ages.

***Types of teeth:***

a) Temporary milk teeth (20)
b) Permanent teeth (32)

***Examination of lower jaw:***

Lower jaw has 2 angles:

**a) Medico-legal angle:** It is obtuse in children, and about a right angle in adults. In old age, it becomes obtuse due to loss of teeth & absorption of alveolar process.

**b) Anatomical angle:** It determines the sex. Mental foramen: It is close to the inferior border in infancy. It is midway between upper and lower border in adults. It comes closer to the upper border in old age due to alveolar process after falling of teeth.

- Stage of ossification of bones & epiphysio - diaphyseal union of long bones:

X-ray is one of the most important factors for the purpose of determination of age. It helps to examine development of union between diaphysis & epiphysis of long bones and ossification of bones. Some other signs for determination of age are: hair in pubic region or axilla, moustache & beard, voice, menstruation, grey hair, wrinkles on the face, etc.

## 18.3 Race, Religion and Sex

***Race:***

Table 18.1 Features of human race

| **Features** | **Mongolian** | **Caucasians** | **Negro** |
|---|---|---|---|
| Complexion | Yellowish | Fair | Black |
| Eyes | Black | Blue | Black |
| Forehead | Inclined forward | Raised | Small |
| Hairs | Straight black | Straight, brown | Thick, curly |
| Face | Large, flat | Small | Prominent molar teeth, projected jaw |
| Nose | Flat | Sharp | Blunt |
| Upper extremity | Small | Normal | Large forearm |
| Lower extremity | Small | Normal | Large leg |

***Religion:*** Describes the values, beliefs and practices related to sacred or spiritual concerns. The study of mutual interactions between the religion and other institutes. It is the organized response of a group of people towards a super – natural power.

***Sex:***

- Sex determination seems easy, but may cause challenges in cases of hermaphrodites, concealed sex, decomposed bodies & skeletal remains.
- The person having varying proportions of both male & female characters is called

***hermaphrodite.***

- Data for identification: Features & facial appearances, length of scalp hair, size & shape of lips, clothes, breast, vagina, uterus, penis, prostate
- To determine true sex: External examination, Examination of internal organs, Gonadal biopsy, Study of sex chromosomes.

Table 18.2 Features of human gender

| Features | Male | Female |
|---|---|---|
| Body hairs | Over chest and limbs | Not significant |
| Hair on pinna | Present | Absent |
| Moustache, beard | Present | Absent |
| Shoulder : Hip | Shoulder broader | Hips broader |
| Thyroid cartilage | Prominent | Not prominent |
| Breast | Rudimentary | Well developed |
| Chest and abdomen | Chest dimensions high | Abdomen dimensions high |
| Waist | Not well defined | Well defined |
| External genitalia | Scrotum, testes, penis | Labia, clitoris, vagina |
| Internal genitalia | Vas deferens, seminal vesicle, prostate | Ovaries, fallopian tubes, uterus |

- **Medico-legal importance of age:** Criminal responsibility, marriage contract, kidnapping, rape, infanticide, criminal abortion, witness competency, eligibility for employment.

## 18.4 Tattoos, Moles, Scars, Occupational marks and Hairs

Tattoo-marks: Design, colour, size & exact anatomical situation of the tattoo should be examined. A tattoo may indicate towards the name of the person or a loved person. It may give suggestion about the person's language. It may give a clue regarding race or religion. Figures of naked women or indecorous female figures indicate the interest of sex.

- **Moles:** Colour, size & exact anatomical situation of the tattoo should be examined.

- **Scars:** A scar is the formation of fibrous tissue as an outcome of the repair process after an injury. It has great value in identification of a person. Following factors of a scar should be examined: Anatomical situation, Size, Shape, Colour, Consistency, and Tenderness.

***Occupational marks:***

1. Temporary marks: Paints, dyes, chemicals or grease at the fingertips of painters, dyers, engineers or mechanics. Microscopic examination of dust or debris under the nail beds or clothes or even in earwax.
2. Permanent marks: Heavy and rough hands are seen in manual labourers. Tailors have needle puncture marks on their left index finger. Thickening of palmer skin in butchers. Copper smelters have greenish hairs. Indigo or cobalt miners have blue hairs.

- **Hairs:** Important in forensic pathology and forensic investigations. Distribution of hair helps to determine gender. Male hairs are thicker and darker than females. Foetus body hair is fine and not pigmented. Grey hairs tend to appear after 30 years in this era. It has greater value of identification in dyeing and bleaching tendency person. Chronic heavy metal poisoning can be detected from hairs. Singeing of the hairs indicates burns. Nature of weapon can be found from injuries to the hairs.

## 18.5 Handwritings, dactylography, DNA typing and Superimposition

- **Handwritings**: Each person has a unique handwriting. Even the identical twins write differently. It helps in identification by: Specific shape of letters, slope of letters, regular or irregular spacing between the letters, rhythmic repetition of the elements, pressure on the paper, average size of the letters, height-width-size of the letters are self-explanatory. Letter comparison, pen lifts, Diacritic placements, connecting strokes, beginning and ending of strokes.

- **Dactylography**: Dactylography is also known as Galton system or Finger Print system. A finger print is the impression of the ball of the finger. It is based on the arrangement of papillary ridges on the skin. No two persons are having identical prints. These prints can easily be taken on paper by ink.

- Types: a) Plain finger print b) Rolled finger print. By the finger print a complete & correct identification of the individual is possible.

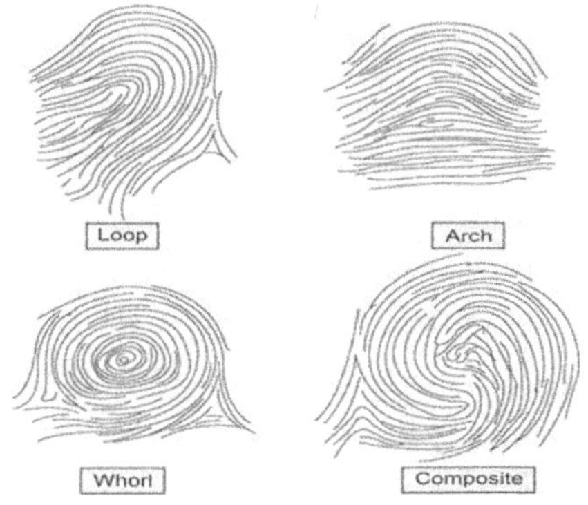

***DNA Profiling:***

**Introduction:** DNA profiling (also called DNA fingerprinting) is the process of determining an individual's DNA characteristics. DNA profiling is a forensic technique in criminal investigations, comparing criminal suspects' profiles to DNA evidence so as to assess the likelihood of their involvement in the crime. Although 99.9% of human DNA sequences are the same in every person, enough of the DNA is different that it is possible to distinguish one individual from another, unless they are monozygotic (identical) twins.

**Process:** The process, developed by Glassberg and independently by Jeffreys, begins with a sample of an individual's DNA (typically called a "reference sample"). Reference samples are usually collected through a buccal swab. When this is unavailable other methods may be needed to collect a sample of blood, saliva, semen, vaginal lubrication, or other fluid or tissue from personal use items or from stored samples. A reference sample is then analysed to create the individual's DNA profile. The DNA profile is then compared against another sample to determine whether there is a genetic match.

**Extraction of DNA:** When a sample such as blood or saliva is obtained, the DNA is only a small part of what is present in the sample. Before the DNA can be analysed, it must be extracted from the cells and purified. There are many ways this can be accomplished, but all methods follow the same basic procedure. The cell and nuclear membranes need to be broken up to allow the DNA to be free in solution. Once the DNA is free, it can be separated from all other cellular components. After the DNA has been separated in solution, the remaining cellular debris can then be removed from the solution and discarded, leaving only DNA. The most common methods of DNA extraction include organic extraction (also called phenol chloroform extraction), Chelex extraction, and solid phase extraction.

**Anthropometry:** The measurements of various parts of the body is called Anthropometry or Bertillon system. It is based on the principle that after the age of 21 years, the skeleton stops growing. Therefore, the measurements of the body parts remain constant and no two persons will have bones of identical dimensions.

- **Disadvantages:** Only applicable to adults, Errors in taking measurements. Many instruments are required for recording the measurements.

***Poroscopy:***

The papillary ridges of the skin of the fingers contain minute pores which are the openings of the ducts of sweat glands. These are permanent and vary in size, shape, portion & number over the given length of ridges in each individual which helps in establishing identity. This method of identification is known as Poroscopy.

***Foot prints:***

Just like a finger print, the foot also gives an impression called as foot print which is useful in identification. The skin patterns of toes & heels are as distinctive as those of the fingers. While examining foot prints, deformities such as web feet, flat feet and supernumerary toes, etc. help in identification of a person.

***Deformities***

Deformities are a burden for the individual, but they are useful for the purpose of identification.

***Types: - 2***

**a) Congenital:** Cleft palate, hare lip, irregular or protruding teeth, moles, supernumerary fingers or toes, flat feet, web feet

**b) Acquired:** Surgical wounds, amputations, mal-united fractures, filling of teeth.

***Miscellaneous data:***

Laundry marks, tailors name marks on clothes, jewels, visiting card, watch, etc. may help in identification of a person.

***Forensic Odontology:***

**Introduction:** Forensic Odontology / Forensic Dentistry is a branch of forensic medicine dealing with teeth and marks left by teeth for identifying criminal suspects or the remains of a dead person. Forensic dentistry is the proper handling, examination and evaluation of dental evidence, which will be then presented in the interest of justice.

***Responsibilities:***

- Forensic dentists are responsible for six main areas of practice:

i. Identification of found human remains
ii. Identification in mass fatalities
iii. Assessment of bite mark injuries
iv. Assessment of cases of abuse
v. Civil cases involving malpractice
vi. Age estimation

The evidence that may be derived from teeth is the age (in children) and identification of the person to whom the teeth belong. This is done by using dental records including radiographs, ante-mortem (prior to death) and post-mortem (after death) photographs and DNA. The other type of evidence is that of bite marks, left on either the victim (by the attacker), the perpetrator (from the victim of an attack), or on an object found at the crime scene.

***Forensic Serology:***

- ***Introduction:***
    - Forensic serology is the detection, identification, classification, and study of various bodily fluids such as blood, semen, saliva, urine, breast milk, vomit,

fecal matter and perspiration, and their relationship to a crime scene.
  - A forensic serologist may also be involved in DNA analysis and bloodstain pattern analysis.
  - Serology testing begins with presumptive tests which gives the analyst an indication that a specific bodily fluid may be present, but cannot completely confirm its presence. Following the presumptive tests, are the confirmatory tests that confirms what the unknown substance actually is.

***Superimposition:***

It is the technique where the post mortem record is kept over the comparable ante mortem record for the comparison. Skull superimposition has 2 phases:

A) Photographic: The ante mortem photograph is enlarged to life size and made as transparent as possible. The anatomic landmarks compared for positive match include: orbits, anterior nasal spine, chin point, angles of the mandible, zygomatic processes. This test helps more in exclusion rather than conclusion.

- **Disadvantage:** A slight change in the enlargement of ante mortem photograph or in angulation can lead to a mismatch.

B) Video: The skull is filmed with video camera 1 and is presented on TV. The facial photograph is then reproduced on the TV monitor with video camera 2. The individual video signals are fed into a vision mixer so that horizontal-vertical wiping, superimposition and negative stimulation can be done. By adjusting the mixer, the video picture of the ante mortem photograph can be enlarged based on the visibility of the vertical facial height.

- **Advantages:** Immediate results, can be videotaped for the court purposes.

C) Facial composite: Graphical representation of an eye witness's memory of a face as recorded by a composite artist.

- **Uses:** Identifying the suspect in a wanted poster, additional evidence against a suspect, warning vulnerable population against serial offenders.

**Multiple Choice Questions**

**1. Which is not a factor for personal identity ?**

A) Race B) Age C) Sex D) Location

**2. DNA profiles is also called as ?**

A) DNA Fingerprinting B) DNA Examination
C) Both D) None

**3. Which of the following is not a congenital deformity ?**

A) Hare lip B) Flat feet
C) Mal – union fracture D) Moles

**4. Name the branch of forensic medicine dealing with teeth ?**

A) DNA Profiling B) Age estimation
C) Anthropometry D) Forensic Odontology

**5. Which identify method uses the papillary ridges on skin having minute pores ?**

A) Poroscopy B) Foot prints
C) Tattoo marks D) Dactylography

**6. Which identified method is also called as Galton method ?**

A) Dactylography B) Poroscopy
C) Anthropometry D) DNA profile

**7. What is the number of temporary teeth ?**

A) 25 B) 20 C) 32 D) 28

**8. Which of the following is not a factor to determine true sex?**

A) Examination of internal organs
B) Gonadal biopsy
C) Study of sex chromosomes
D) Facial features

**9. Which method for personal identification is called as Bertillon System?**

A) Poroscopy
B) Anthropometry
C) Dactylography
D) Odontology

**10. Which of the following is not a shape of fingerprints ?**

A) Loop B) Whorl C) Square D) Arch

**Answer key for MCQs:**

| 1 | D |
|---|---|
| 2 | A |
| 3 | C |
| 4 | D |
| 5 | A |

| 6 | A |
|---|---|
| 7 | B |
| 8 | D |
| 9 | B |
| 10 | C |

# Ch. 19
# Thanatology

## 19.1 Death:

- **Thanatology:** The branch of science which deals with death in all the aspects. It denotes death of human being according to IPC section 46.
- **Definition:** The process in which cellular metabolic process in different tissues and organs cease to function at different rates.

Table 19.1 Types of death

| **Somatic death** | **Molecular death** |
|---|---|
| -Complete and irreversible stoppage of circulation, respiration and brain functions. | -Occurs after Somatic death causing death of all individual cells. |
| -There is stopped aerobic process. | -Aerobic process stops due to non-availability of ATP. |
| -Flat EEG, brain function stops, permanent complete cessation of heart, complete stoppage of lung functions. | -Muscles and pupils do not respond to stimuli. |
| -Muscles and pupils respond to external stimuli. | -Early signs:<br>-Changes in skin and eye, body cools down, post-mortem lividity, muscles relaxation. |
| -Criteria for brain death:<br>-Stimuli don't produce any response except deep tendon reflex which are intact.<br>-Absent pupillary reflex, corneal reflex, pharyngeal and tracheal reflex.<br>-Apnoea and absent response to atropine. | -Late signs:<br>-Putrefaction, adipocere formation and mummification. |

***Medico-legal importance of death:***

- Declaration of death has importance for cremation and burial.
- Certification of death, disposal of body.
- Organ transplantation cannot be done till there is certification of death. Use of tissue for transplant can be done only after this.
- Presumption of death.

***Mode of death:***

Table 19.2

| Coma | Asphyxia | Syncope |
|---|---|---|
| -It is the state of complete unconsciousness. | -A state of acute lack of oxygen in living organism along with inability to remove excess carbon dioxide. | -Stoppage of function of heart with continuous cessation of circulation. |
| -Person characterized by complete insensibility | -Mechanical: Hanging, strangulation, throttling, drowning.<br>-Pathologic: Consolidation, pleural effusion. | -There is loss of consciousness and postural collapse due to acute decrease in cerebral blood flow. |
| -No response to external stimuli. | Toxic: Opium, CO, Cyanide poisoning. | -Causes: Myocardial infarction, stenosis, pulmonary hypertension, anaemia. |
| -Causes:<br>Head injury, intracranial haemorrhage, encephalitis, meningitis, diabetic ketoacidosis, hepatic encephalopathy, opium poisoning. | -Pathologic: Consolidation, pleural effusion.<br>-Environmental: High altitude, trapped in a well, respiration in a closed room. | |

***Suspended animation:***

- A condition of living body in which all activities characteristic of life are temporarily suspended giving appearance of death.

- Condition lasts for ½ hour or more.
- May be found in electrocution, drowning, after anaesthesia, stroke, narcotic poisoning, new-born infants.

***Post-mortem changes after death:***

1. Immediate response:
    - Stoppage of nervous system function
    - Stoppage of respiration
    - Stoppage of circulation

2. Early changes:
    - Changes in skin
    - Changes in eyes
    - Changes in body
    - Post-mortem lividity
    - Rigor mortis
    - Changes in body fluids

3. Later changes:
    - Putrefaction
    - Adipocere
    - Mummification

## 19.2 Signs of death:

***1. Immediate signs due to somatic death:***

A. Permanent and complete cessation of functions for long:

- Stoppage of breathing for more than 5 minutes leading to no breathing sounds in larynx.

Table 19.3 Tests confirming cessation of breath

| | |
|---|---|
| **Feather test** | No movement of feather when held in front of nose |
| **Mirror test** | Mirror held in front of nose shows no vapour and blurring |
| **Winslow's test** | No movement seen when mirror kept on chest |

B. Permanent and complete cessation of functions of heart and ECG:

- There is completed Stoppage and flat ECG for 3 minutes.

Table 19.4 Tests confirming cessation of circulation

| | |
|---|---|
| **Magnus test** | Fingers fail to show congestion and swelling when ligature applied at base. |
| **Diaphanous test** | Finger web spaces fail to show redness on trans-illumination. |
| **Icard's test** | Failure of yellowish green discoloration on injecting flurescin dye. |
| **Finger nail test** | No filling of blood seen on applying and releasing pressure. |

***2. Early signs of death:***

A. Skin: Loss of translucency and elasticity. Skin becomes greyish white, lips becomes brown and hard.

B. Eye: Abolition of pupillary and corneal reflexes. Cornea becomes hazy and white. Cellular debris and mucous form yellow triangle at each of cornea. Decrease in IOP leading to flaccidity of eye. There is increase in potassium, ascorbic acid and lactic acid in vitreous humour.

C. Algorithm mortis

D. Livor mortis

E. Muscular changes: Primary relaxation, Algorithm mortis, secondary relaxation.

***Algor Mortis:***

- Algor mortis is the post-mortem cooling of the body. After death, heat is transferred from the body to a solid surface, fluid, or into the air via the physical processes of conduction, radiation, or convection. Cooling will continue at a certain rate until the body reaches the ambient temperature.
- The rate of cooling occurs much more rapidly with immersion

in cold water. Since the skin is the closest to the air, cooling occurs more rapidly there, and thus the measurement of the core temperature gives a better representation of the body's temperature.

- The core body temperature can be measured by either placing a thermometer through a small incision of the upper right abdominal quadrant into the liver or inserting the thermometer into the rectum.
- Initial 45 minutes: no temperature change (isothermic phase).
    - 1 – 6 hours: 1.5° to 2° C/hr
    - 6 – 12 hours: 0.9° to 1.20° C/hr
    - After 24 hours: 0.4° to 0.6° C/hr
- Generally, temperature change is considered an inaccurate means of determining time of death, as the rate of change is affected by several key factors:
- Stability or fluctuation of the ambient temperature.
- The thickness and body coverage of clothing or similar materials.
- Diseases or drugs which increase body temperature and thereby raise the starting temperature of the corpse at the time of death.

***Livor Mortis:***

- Livor mortis starts within 20–30 minutes, but is usually not observable by the human eye until two hours after death. The size of the patches increases in the next three to six hours.
- Fixation will begin to occur during this timeframe, causing the patches to be unaltered due to movement.
- Maximum lividity will occur between eight and twelve hours after death.
- Areas of blood pooling in contact with the ground will blanch, or remain white.
- The blood pools into the interstitial tissues of the body. The intensity of the colour depends upon the amount of reduced

haemoglobin in the blood.

- The discoloration does not occur in the areas of the body that are in contact with the ground or another object, in which capillaries are compressed.

***Rigor Mortis:***

- Rigor mortis is initially apparent in small muscles, such as the muscles of the hands and face, which become noticeably stiff within three to four hours after death.
- In some instances, immediate muscle relaxation and rigor mortis-induced fixation upon death causes an open-eyed grimacing facial expression.
- Larger muscles are affected later, usually around 12 hours, leading to stiffening of the entire body.
- Rigor mortis results from the cessation of breathing and oxygen intake following death, which leads to the termination of aerobic respiration, the main process by which cells generate energy in the form of adenosine triphosphate (ATP).
- In rigor mortis and the absence of ATP, however, myosin is unable to change its conformation to dissociate from actin, and muscles remain in a contracted, stiffened state. Other chemical characteristics of rigor mortis include the accumulation of lactic acid in muscle tissue and post-mortem leakage of calcium ions into the sarcomere, where myosin and actin filaments are located.
- Lactic acid is produced post-mortem as still-living muscle cells switch from aerobic to anaerobic metabolism; as lactic acid builds up inside cells during rigor, it causes a decrease in pH levels.
- Stage 1: In the absent stage, the body is still relaxed, and its parts can be moved into different positions.
- Stage 2: As rigor mortis progresses from minimal to complete, the body becomes increasingly stiff.
- Stage 3: with parts remaining in their positions until the passed

phase, when the muscles begin to lose their stiffness and liver mortis and decay set in.

**MARCH OF RIGOR: It takes 12 hours to occur Rigor mortis, it remains for another 12 hours and completed in next 12 hours.**

***Adipocere:***

- Adipocere is also known as corpse wax, grave wax.
- Formed by the anaerobic bacterial hydrolysis of fat in tissue, such as body fat in cadavers.
- Pale, rancid greasy fluid with unpleasant smell.
- When fully formed it becomes grey and waxy.

***Skeletalization:***

- Due to autolysis or being eaten by animals.
- In a firmly buried body, tissues will be absent in 2 years.
- On examination of bone marrow space, it shows residual organic matter which is suitable for DNA analysis.

***Mummification:***

- Mummification is a modification of the putrefaction process.
- It is characterized by the desiccation or dehydration of the cadaveric tissues.
- The skin of the deceased becomes brown, hard, and brittle and has a stretched appearance over prominences like the zygomatic bones, mandible.
- The time it takes for a body to mummify depends on the body's size and conditions, but it usually takes several weeks to months.
- Mummification can occur in extremely dry environments, such as ancient Egypt.
- It can also occur in non-desert conditions, occasionally in new-born infants, and rarely in adults in hot and dry climates.
- A mummified body has dark, tightly adhered skin, a parchment-

like appearance, and no smell.

- The internal organs get converted into dried, shrivelled up masses.

***Death certificate:***

- The medical examiner or coroner is responsible for filling out a death certificate in cases where a crime or foul play is suspected.
- The attending physician usually fills out the medical portion of the death certificate based on their assessment.
- According to Registration of Birth and Death act 1969: The Medical officer informs the registrar about the birth or death in the hospital [Section 8 (b)].
- The certificate will be issued without charging any fee [Section 10 (3)].
- Any Registered Medical Practitioner who denies or neglects to give the certificate under Sub-section 3 of Section 10 of the Registration of Birth and Death act 1969, will be punished with fine which may extend up to Rs 50.

Table 19.5

| | |
|---|---|
| Cause of death | The immediate cause of death, which can be a disease, clinical condition, or event that made life unsustainable. |
| Manner of death | Whether the death was natural, accidental, homicidal, suicidal, or indeterminable. |
| Circumstances of death | Dates, places, and how the injury occurred, if applicable. |
| Certifier | The name and title of the certifier. |
| Access | The death certificate is a public record that can be accessed by the family, lawyers, insurance companies, and clinical researchers. |
| Importance | Death certificates are vital records that help track the health of populations, identify health hazards, and inform public health policies and healthcare practices. |

## 19. 3 Medico-legal autopsy and exhumation:

***Autopsy:***

- A medico-legal autopsy is a post-mortem examination performed to establish the cause of death or other relevant factors in cases that are suspicious, unnatural, or sudden.
- The results of a medico-legal autopsy can be used as evidence in legal proceedings such as criminal trials, civil suits, and administrative hearings.

Table 19.6

| | |
|---|---|
| Who performs it | A recognized medical officer, usually at the request of a police officer or magistrate. |
| When it's performed | In cases of sudden, unnatural, or suspicious deaths. |
| What it involves | A systematic examination of the body to determine the cause, manner, and time of death. |
| What's collected | Fingernail scrapings, swabs, and clippings, saliva samples, and photographs of injuries. |

***Types:***

1. Forensic:

- To identify the decent and to find out the manner of death.
- Done in cases such as violent death, unnatural death or death without medical assistance.

2. Medical:

- To diagnose a specific disease for research purposes.
- Example: material for infectious disease can be collected to study or research on it.
- The aim is to clarify the medical diagnosis which remained unknown.

3. Anatomical:

- Performed by the students of anatomy only for the purpose of study.

4. Virtual:

- Done using the imagining techniques: only MRI, CT.

***Exhumation:***

- Exhumation is the process of removing a body or cremated remains from the ground, or disturbing remains within a grave.
- It's a rare process that's usually only permitted in exceptional circumstances.

***The reasons include:***

- Repatriation: To return the deceased to their country of origin
- Cremation: To fulfil the deceased's wishes, which may have been discovered after burial
- Lack of burial space: To make room for new burials
- Redevelopment: To make way for redevelopment of a cemetery or crypt
- Archaeological reasons: For research purposes
- Criminal investigations: To aid in criminal investigations
- Incorrect burial: To correct an error, such as burying the deceased in the wrong plot.
- Exhumations can be challenging because of a number of factors, including:
- Post-mortem toxicology investigations are rare, enzymes can affect drug concentrations, autolysis can release exogenous compounds, and bacteria metabolism can affect toxicological analysis results.
- Uses: To reach identification; such in the case of missing persons or human remains of victims of terrorist attacks, major catastrophes, mass graves or armed conflicts.

## 19.4 The Transplantation of Human Organs and Tissues Act:

- The Transplantation of Human Organs & Tissues Act (THOTA), 1994 provides for regulation of removal, storage and transplantation of human organs & tissues for therapeutic purposes and for prevention of commercial dealings in human organs & tissues.

- The Government of India has implemented National Organ Transplant Program (NOTP) to establish a network of organ and tissue transplant organizations at national, regional and state level.
- This act is applicable to only those Indian administered states where the act has been adopted or enforced by the state governments. But it applies to all Union territories.

***Objectives:***

- The primary objectives of the Transplantation of Human Organs and Tissues Act, 1994 is to prevent commercial and illegal donations or advertisements of human organs.
- Any person whether they are transplantation coordinator, or associated to any medical college or hospital or those who helps in removing of human organ or tissues from an alive or deceased body without any authority, shall be imprisoned for the term of three years with a fine of 5 lakh rupees.
- The Act contains detailed provisions relating to the authority for removal of human organs, preservation of human organs, regulation of hospitals conducting the removal, storage or transplantation of human organs.
- Brain Stem death is recognized as a legal death in India under the Transplantation of Human Organs and Tissues Act.
- After natural cardiac death only a few organs/tissues can be donated (like cornea, bone, skin and blood vessels) whereas after brain stem death almost 8-9 organs including vital organs.
- Some of the important amendments under this Act to promote organ donation are as follows.
- Provision of 'Retrieval Centres' for retrieval of organs from deceased donors and their registration under the amended Act.
- Definition of near relative expanded to include grandparents and grandchildren.

- Swap Donation (Donor Exchange) included.
- Brain death certification Board has been simplified and more experts have been permitted for this certification.
- 'Mandatory' inquiry and informing option to donate in case of unfortunate event of brain stem death of ICU patient for the purpose of organ donation.
- Mandatory 'Transplant Coordinator' for coordinating all matters relating to removal or transplantation of human organs.
- National Human Organs and Tissues Removal and Storage Network at one or more places and regional network.
- National Registry of Donors and Recipients.
- Removal of eye has been permitted by a trained technician to facilitate eye donation.
- To protect vulnerable and poor there is provision of higher penalties has been made for trading in organs (imprisonment up to 10 years and fine up to Rs
- One crore).
- Act has made provision of greater caution in case of minors and foreign nationals and prohibition of organ donation from mentally challenged persons

**Multiple Choice Questions**

**1. Thanatology defined under which section of IPC.**

A. 40 B. 46 C. 51 D. 66

**2. WBC die after what duration of cardiac arrest?**

A. 05 B. 08 C. 12 D. 15

**3. Which of the following does not come under the early signs of death?**

A. Eye changes B. Skin changes
C. Putrefaction D. Body fluids

**4. How many types of autopsy are mentioned?**

A. 4 B. 6 C. 8 D. 10

**5. The internal organs get converted into dried, shrivelled up masses in which of the following?**

A. Putrefaction B. Mummification

C. Skeletalization D. Adipocere

**6. The post-mortem cooling of the body is known as?**

A. Rigor mortis B. Algor mortis

C. Livor mortis D. Putrefaction

**7. No movement of feather when held in front of nose?**

A. Mirror test B. Feather test

C. Diaphanous test D. Winslow's test

**8. Initially apparent in small muscles, which become noticeably stiff within three to four hours after death is called?**

A. Mummification B. Livor mortis

C. Algor mortis D. Rigor mortis

**9. Failure of yellowish green discoloration on injecting flurescin dye?**

A. Icard's test B. Feather test

C. Feather test D. Magnus test

**10. Virtual autopsy is done by which technique?**

A. MRI B. USG C. X-ray D. PET scan

**Answer key for MCQs:**

| | |
|---|---|
| 1 | B |
| 2 | C |
| 3 | C |
| 4 | A |
| 5 | B |

| | |
|---|---|
| 6 | B |
| 7 | B |
| 8 | D |
| 9 | A |
| 10 | A |

# Ch. 20
# Asphyxial Deaths

## 20.1 Hanging:

***Definition:***

- A lack of oxygen or excess of carbon dioxide in the body that results in unconsciousness and often death.
- Is usually caused by interruption of breathing or inadequate oxygen supply.
- Identified by: Cyanosis, congestion, tardieu's spots.

***Types:***

- Hanging
- Suffocation
- Strangulation
- Drowning

***1. Hanging:***

- Caused by the suspension of body by a ligature around the neck where the constricting force being weight of body.

Table 20.1 Types of hanging

| Complete | Incomplete | Typical | Atypical |
|---|---|---|---|
| Body is fully suspended and no part of body touches ground. | Partial suspension and some part of body touches ground. | Ligature is in midline above the thyroid cartilage symmetrical upward on both sides of neck. | Knot being other than occiput or nape of neck. |
| Constricting force is weight of body. | Constricting force being the head. | The point of suspension being on occiput. | Most common site being in near one side of mastodon process or mandible. |

***Causes of death in hanging:***

- Cerebral ischemia and anoxia due to compression of carotid artery.
- Cerebral congestion due to compression of jugular veins.
- Asphyxia due to compression of airways.
- Neurogenic shock and fracture dislocation of upper cervical vertebrae with damage to spinal cord.

***Important post-mortem finding:***

- Ligature mark over thyroid cartilage directed obliquely upwards towards mandible then to mastoid and finally to occipital protuberance.
- Under ligature, there is dry - white and glistening pad of fat.
- Dribbling of saliva from the angle of mouth which confirms ante-mortem hanging.
- Intimate tear of carotid artery.
- In case of ligature pressure on cervical sympathetic ganglia. The eye on that side is found open.
- Tardieu spots are not as profound in strangulation.

***Ligature marks:***

- Pressure mark on the neck under the ligature.
- Common injury in hanging and strangulation.

Table 20.2

| **Fixed noose** | **Running noose** |
|---|---|
| Rope is tied around the neck to tie a fixed knot. | One end of the rope is passed through the loop made from the other end. |
| Ligature mark is inverted V-shape. | Ligature mark is horizontal shape. |

***Judicial hanging:***

- In India, the legal death sentence given by hanging the

criminal.
- Placement of knot beneath the chin is used mostly.
- The person is allowed to drop 5-7 meters according to weight.
- Sudden Stoppage causes fracture dislocation of C2-C3 or C3-C4 vertebrae causing injury to brainstem and spinal cord.

***Lynching:***
- Homicidal hanging where a person accused is killed by a group of people.
- The name is derived from Willaim Lynch, a white captain in USA who used to give order to hand the blacks without any trials.

***Sexual asphyxia:***
- Also known as auto-erotic asphyxia.
- Sexual asphyxia is almost always practiced by males during solitary sexual activity especially in the mid-20s.
- Bodies found at the scene of an accidental death may show evidence of other paraphilic activities, such as fetishistic cross-dressing and masochism.

## 20.2 Strangulation and Suffocation

***1. Strangulation :***
- The act of compressing the neck, which can lead to asphyxia and neuronal death.
- The force constricting is external.

***Signs of strangulation:***
- Redness
- Scratches or abrasions
- Fingernail impressions in the skin
- Deep fingernail claw marks
- Ligature marks
- Thumbprint-shaped bruises

- Blood-red eyes
- Pinpoint red spots

***Types of strangulation:***

Table 20.3

| Ligature | Throttling | Bansdola | Garroting | Mugging |
|---|---|---|---|---|
| Neck is tied with a ligature. | Neck is compressed by 1 or 2 hands. | Compression of neck done suddenly. | Compression of neck with rope from behind. | Also known as chock hold. |
| Multiple rounds of ligature given with no knots. | When compressed with palms, it is palmar throttling. | Substance used are bamboo stick or wooden sticks. | Spanish windlass is garroting where iron cotton is tied around neck with a screw. | Compression of neck by forearm or a fold in elbow. |

***Important post-mortem finding of strangulation:***

There is a complete continuous ligature mark below thyroid. The mark is horizontal.

- The mark area is haemorrhagic with lacerated blood vessels.
- Strangulation is more violent than hanging, usually causing more damage.
- Hyoid bone fracture occurs and laryngeal along with tracheal structures are damaged.
- Subcutaneous tissue and muscle damage in neck.
- No saliva dribbling from mouth and cervical vertebrae fracture.
- Multiple petechial haemorrhage and haemorrhagic eyes.
- Tongue is swollen, protruded and bitten.
- Possible incontinence.
- Congested internal organs with multiple haemorrhage.

## *Difference between Hanging and Strangulation:*

| Features | Hanging | Strangulation |
|---|---|---|
| Suspension of body | Present | Absent |
| Neck compression | Caused by ligature, knee or foot. | Caused by ligature, hands, stick or elbow. |
| Force of compression | Endogenous force | Exogenous force |
| Ligature | Above the thyroid, oblique, symmetric and incomplete. | On or below thyroid, horizontal continuous complete. |
| Knot | Usually present | Usually absent |
| Knot site mark | Usually absent | Not applicable |
| Mark shape | Inverted V shaped in fix knot. | Multiple ligature marks. |
| Mark surface | Contused, pattern of ligature used visible. | Haemorrhagic and soft due to bleeding. |
| Surface hardness | Hard | Soft |
| Blood vessels | Usually no laceration | Lacerated |
| Vertebrae | C2-C3 or C3-C4 fractured. | No fracture |
| Hyoid bone fracture | Not common | Occurs specially in throttling |
| Spinal cord injury | Spinal cord, pons, medulla injured. | No such injuries. |
| Struggle marks | Not found as most cases are suicidal. | Contusion and laceration marks present. |
| Sexual assault | Rare in female victims. | May be a part of sexual assault. |
| Concealment of crime | Usually not done. | Body may be burnt or disposed in jungle. |
| Head tilt | Found on knot side | No tilting |
| Neck appearance | Stretched | Not stretched |
| Face appearance | Pale | Congested and deeply cyanosed. |
| Cyanosis | Mild cyanosis of lips, nose, ear, nail. | Severe cyanosis |
| Petechial haemorrhage | Few found on eyes, nails. | Multiple with protruded eyes. |

| Tongue | Usually inside | Protruded bitten and black. |
|---|---|---|
| Saliva dribbling | Present at the angle of mouth | Usually absent. |

***2. Suffocation:***

- A form of asphyxia caused by blocking air entry into the respiratory tract but not due to compression and drowning.
- It includes smothering, gagging, choking, traumatic asphyxia.

| Smothering | Blocking the nose and mouth preventing air entry. Done using hands, cloth or plastic bag. |
|---|---|
| Choking | Caused by internal blockage of the airway like food stuck in throat obstructing glottis. |
| Gagging | A type of choking where airway is blocked by placing a piece of cloth or object inside the mouth and nostrils. |
| Traumatic asphyxia | Caused by mechanical compression of chest preventing normal breathing due to blunt trauma to chest, back or abdomen. Leads to respiratory arrest.<br>Eg: Stampede, crush injuries from road accident. |
| Burking | Combination of smothering and chest asphyxia. Historically used by Burk and Hare. One would sit on chest and block nose and mouth while other would drag the body. |
| Cafe coronary | Sudden death caused by choking on bolus of food that obstructs the larynx. More common in elderly and depressed gag reflex due to tranquilizers.<br>Ex: Mechanical asphyxia<br>Reflex cardiac arrest. |
| Over lying | A form of asphyxia where external compression of chest obstruct normal respiration.<br>Ex: Bed sharing with infant. |

## 20.3 Drowning

- Drowning is a type of asphyxial death that occurs when the entry of air into the lungs is blocked by water or another fluid entering the respiratory passages through the nose and mouth.
- For drowning to cause death, the nose and mouth must be

submerged in water. However, it is not necessary for the entire body to be underwater.

***Types of drowning:***

1. Typical Drowning
2. Atypical Drowning

***Typical drowning:***

- In typical drowning, water or another fluid enters the airways and lungs, leading to obstruction of air passages. This is why it's called "wet drowning."
- During post-mortem examination, fluid and froth are typically found in the airways and lungs.

**A) Fresh water drowning:**

- A large amount of water enters the bloodstream through the alveolar membranes.
- This leads to hypervolemia (increased blood volume) and hemodilution (dilution of blood).
- Red blood cells absorb the water and burst (a process called hemolysis), releasing potassium.
- The heart experiences volume overload and an excess of potassium.
- There is also a sodium deficit (known as hyponatremia) and a lack of oxygen (anoxia).
- The combination of anoxia and hyperkalemia (high potassium levels) can lead to ventricular fibrillation (a life-threatening heart rhythm disturbance).
- Death usually occurs within 4–5 minutes.

**B) Salt water drowning:**

- The inhaled water is hypertonic (has a high salt concentration).
- Rapid development of pulmonary edema, accompanied by progressively worsening low blood volume (hypovolemia).

- Onset of circulatory shock.
- Eventually, the heart stops (asystole), leading to death within 8 to 12 minutes.

**Atypical Drowning:**

- In atypical drowning, little or no water enters the respiratory passages or lungs, even though the body is submerged. Froth and water are generally not found in the lungs.
- Atypical drowning can occur in the following forms:

***A) Dry drowning:***

- When a person comes in contact with water, especially cold water, it may trigger a strong laryngospasm (spasm of the vocal cords), which prevents water from entering the lungs.
- Death occurs due to asphyxia caused by this laryngospasm.

***B) Immersion Syndrome:***

- This condition causes sudden death due to vagal inhibition triggered by:
- A sudden splash of cold water
- Duck diving (falling feet-first into water)

***C) Unconscious submersion:***

- Unconsciousness may be due to stroke, heart attack, epilepsy, hypertension.
- If the person is already unconscious before entering the water, little or no water gets into the respiratory tract.

***D) Near drowning:***

- In near drowning, the person initially survives the drowning event but later dies due to complications.
- This may happen after the person is rescued from water, either conscious or unconscious.
- Death occurs later as a result of hypoxic encephalopathy

(brain damage due to lack of oxygen) and fibrosing alveolitis (scarring of lung tissue).

**Important post-mortem finding of drowning:**

***A) External findings:***

- The eyes are typically open, with dilated pupils.
- The conjunctiva appears congested, and there may be small hemorrhages present.
- The skin often shows cutis anserina (goose skin) due to contraction of the small muscles (erector pili).
- The hands and feet may appear white, wrinkled, and corrugated, especially in people who drowned while performing water-related tasks like washing clothes.
- There is usually a white, fine, lathery, and abundant froth, which becomes more prominent when the chest is compressed.
- The froth is usually not blood-tinged, and it is more abundant and persistent than in poisonings.
- Victims often clutch weeds, grass, mud, or stones in their hands due to a cadaveric spasm.
- Abraded tips of fingers, toes, and sand under nails may also be found but have limited forensic value.
- Post-mortem lividity is light pink or violet seen on face, upper chest and hands.

***B) Internal findings:***

- The air passages contain white, fine, lathery, and sticky froth.
- The lungs may show subpleural hemorrhages, often called Paltauf's hemorrhages.
- Petechial hemorrhages may also be present.
- Emphysema aquosa found only in wet drowning.

***C) Specific signs:***

- Water in the stomach and intestines.The presence of water in the stomach and intestines indicates that the person was alive at the time of drowning. This is because, in postmortem drowning, water may be present in the esophagus but not beyond the cardiac sphincter.

- After putrefaction, relaxation of the cardiac and pyloric sphincters occurs, making the presence of water in the stomach and intestines insignificant in such cases.
- Diatoms found in the brain and bone marrow are also diagnostic and even more significant than water in the stomach and intestines—especially in decomposed (putrefied) bodies, as diatoms resist putrefaction.
- The diatom test is negative in cases where dead bodies are thrown into water or in dry drowning.

***D) Gettler test:***

- The Gettler test is used to determine drowning as the cause of death.
- It estimates the chloride content of blood in both chambers of the heart. Normally, the chloride level is equal in the right and left chambers, approximately 600 mg/100 ml.
- In freshwater drowning, hemodilution occurs, decreasing the chloride content.
- In saltwater drowning, hemoconcentration leads to an increased chloride content in the left side of the heart.
- A 25% difference in chloride levels between the two sides of the heart is considered significant.

**Limitations of the Gettler Test:**

***1. Limited Use in Atypical Drowning Cases:***

The test has no value in atypical drowning scenarios, such as cases involving congenital heart defects (e.g., cardiac shunts or a patent foramen ovale), or if the drowning medium contains the same chloride concentration as blood.

***2. Postmortem Changes:***

There is a progressive loss of chloride ions from blood after death. Therefore, the Gettler test must be conducted within a reasonably short time after death to yield reliable results.

- Suicidal Drowning:
  - Indicated by the absence of struggle or assault signs (e.g., no torn clothing or injury marks).
  - In cases of determined suicide, individuals may tie their hands and legs together, attach weights to their body, consume poison, or cut their throat before immersion.

- Homicidal Drowning:
  - Shows clear signs of violence or struggle (e.g., head injuries, marks of strangulation, or throttling).
  - The head and feet may be tied, or heavy objects may be fastened to the body, or the body might be placed inside a gunny bag.
  - Homicidal drowning is rare, usually observed in infants or children.

- Accidental Drowning:
  - This is the most common type of drowning.
  - Typically seen in children, non-swimmers, or during floods, or when a person accidentally falls into a well, etc.

**Multiple Choice Questions**

**1. Which of the following is not a type of hanging?**

A. Partial B. Typical C. Incomplete D. Atypical

**2. In fixed noose what is the shape of ligature mark?**

A. Inverted S B. Inverted U

C. Inverted V D. Inverted L

**3. In hanging which vertebrae is fractured?**

A. C3 B. C1 C. T10 D. L5

**4. Compression of neck with rope from behind is called**

A. Mugging B. Throttling

C. Garroting D. Bansdola

**5. Tongue is protruded bitten and black in**

A. Hanging B. Suffocation

C. Drowning D. Strangulation

**Answer key for MCQs:**

| | |
|---|---|
| 1. | A |
| 2. | C |
| 3. | A |
| 4. | C |
| 5. | D |

# Ch. 21
# Injury

## 21.1 Basics of injury:

***Definition:***

- Injury means damage to any part of the body caused by mechanical force.
- Legal Definition: Any internal or external harm caused by violence, with or without breaking the skin.
- As per Section 44 of IPC, injury is "any harm caused illegally to a person's body, mind, reputation, or property."

**Classification of injuries:**

***A) Mechanical injury:***

1. Blunt force injury:
- Abrasions
- Laceration
- Contusion
- Fracture

2. Sharp edge injuries:
- Incised wounds
- Cut wounds

3. Piercing injury:
- Stab wounds

4. Firearm injury:
- Gunshot injury

***B) Thermal injury:***

1. Due to cold:

- Frost bite
- Trench foot
- Immersion foot

2. Due to heat:

- Burns
- Scales

***C) Chemical injuries:***

- Corrosion
- Irritation

***D) Miscellaneous injury:***

- Electricity
- X-rays
- Lightening
- Radio active substance

***E) Medico-legal injury:***

- Suicidal injury
- Homicidal injury
- Accidental wounds
- Fabricated wounds
- Defence wounds

***F) Injuries in relation to death:***

- Antemortem injury
- Postmortem injury

***G) Legal classification:***

- Simple injury
- Grievous injury

*Abrasion:*

- An abrasion is a mechanical injury where the outermost skin layer (epidermis) or mucous membrane is scraped off due to rubbing against a rough surface.

**Types of abrasion:**

***1. Linear abrasion:***

- Also called scratch abrasion.
- Caused by sharp, narrow objects like a pin, thorn, nail, barb, prickle, or pointed weapon tip.

***2. Graze abration:***

- Occurs when the skin slides over a rough surface.
- It appears wider at the starting point and narrows at the end.
- Characterized by uneven, longitudinal, parallel marks.

***3. Pressure abration:***

- Caused by continuous pressure from an object.
- Example: Mark on the skin due to pressure from an object like rope or blunt edge.

***4. Imprint abration:***

- The shape or pattern of the object causing the injury is imprinted on the skin.
- Example: Injury marks from sticks, rods, or similar shaped items.

***5. Tire Mark abration:***

- Seen in road traffic accidents.
- Appears as patterns of vehicle parts over the skin.

***Medico-legal importance:***

- Helps determine the site of impact and direction of applied force.

- Can help identify the type of weapon/object used.
- Age of the injury can help establish the time of assault.
- Most abrasions are simple injuries, but if the eye (cornea) is involved, it may cause permanent vision damage, making it a grievous injury.
- May provide clues about the type of offense committed.

**Contusion:**

- Collection of blood because of blood vessel rupture by applying mechanical force in continuity is contusion .

***Types:***

- Intradermal bruise
- Subcutaneous bruise
- Patterned contusion
- Deep bruise
- Tram-line contusion
- Six-penny bruises
- Horse-shoe-shaped contusion
- Contusion over organs
- Gravitating or shifting contusion
- Spectacle hematoma

***Bruises:***

- Leakage of blood into tissues from damaged blood vessels.
- Yellow color usually appears after 18 hours.
- Conditions for bruise:

1.Injury to small blood vessels.
2. Blood leaks into skin or deeper tissues.

***Medico-legal importance:***

- Offending weapon can be identified.
- Age of the injury can be estimated.

- Nature and manner of injury (accidental/homicidal/suicidal) can be known.
- Degree of violence can be evaluated.

***Laceration:***

- A mechanical injury caused by blunt force leading to splitting or tearing of skin and tissue.
- Looks like cuts, splits, or tears.
- Often bleeds and may have bruising or abrasions at edges.
- Scalp, face, elbows, knees, shins are common sites.

***Types of laceration:***

1. Split Laceration – Looks like an incised wound but caused by blunt force.
2. Stretch Laceration – Skin tears due to over-stretching.
3. Tear Laceration – Skin and tissue are torn.
4. Avulsion Laceration – Skin gets pulled off from deeper layers.
5. Crush Laceration – Tissue or limb is partially or totally severed.
6. Cut Laceration – Caused by sharp-edged tools (rare, resembles incised wounds.

***Medico-legal importance:***

- Helps identify cause of injury.
- Type of laceration can be known.
- Can determine if injury is simple or grievous.
- Foreign objects in wound help trace weapon or location.
- Age of injury can be estimated.
- Helps identify if injury is suicidal, accidental, or homicidal.
- Direction of force can be determined.
- May look like an incised wound (can be confusing).

***Incised wounds:***

- A type of mechanical injury caused by a sharp object that

cleanly cuts through skin and tissues. The features are:

- Wound is broader than the weapon's edge.
- Length of the wound is more than its depth or width.
- Starting end is deeper than the end point.
- More bleeding (haemorrhage).

***Medico-legal importance:***

- Cause of injury can be identified.
- Nature of injury (simple or grievous) can be known.
- Age of injury can be estimated.
- Whether injury is accidental, suicidal, or homicidal can be assessed.
- Direction of force used can be known.
- May be confused with lacerated wound.
- May be self-inflicted.
- May be defensive injury.
- May be fabricated wound.

***Chop wounds:***

- A type of incised wound made using a heavy and sharp object like an axe, sword, or chopper. The featured are:
- Caused by sharp heavy weapons.
- Wound is wider and deeper than normal incised wounds.

***Medico-legal importance:***

- Usually homicidal.
- Position of the assailant and victim can be determined.
- Type of weapon used can be known.
- Age of the injury can be estimated.

***Stab wounds:***

- A piercing wound caused by pointed or narrow objects along the long axis of the weapon.

*Types:*

1. Puncture Wound – Depth is the greatest.
2. Penetrating Wound – Object enters body (e.g. chest, abdomen).
3. Perforating Wound – Object passes completely through.
4. Concealed Puncture Wound – Not easily visible.

***Medico-legal importance:***

- Can be suicidal, homicidal, or accidental.
- Type and size of weapon can be identified.
- Movement of weapon inside the wound can be known.
- Depth and direction of wound can be known.
- Force applied can be estimated.
- Age of the wound can be determined.
- Manner of injury (suicidal, homicidal, accidental) can be known.

**Other types of injury:**

***1. Punching:***

- A blow with a clenched fist.
- Usually seen on bony parts like face or skull.
- May result in abrasions, bruises, lacerations, fractures.
- Face/mouth injury may need internal (intraoral) examination.

***2. Kicking and Stamping:***

- Injuries from foot impact, often to face, chest, or abdomen.
- Can cause internal organ damage.

***3. Bite Injuries:***

- Seen in sexual assaults, child abuse, or sports.

***4. Defence injury:***

- Occur when a person tries to protect themselves from an attack using hands and arms, especially against sharp weapons.
- Common site: arm and hand

*5. Self inflicted injury:*

- Injuries a person inflicts on themselves, often seen in suicide attempts or to fake an attack. The features are:
- May be blunt or sharp force injuries.
- Found at "elective sites":
- Sharp force (cuts): wrists and neck.
- Stab wounds: chest and abdomen.
- Injuries are often multiple, parallel, and superficial.
- Bite marks may also be present on arms.

*6. Torture injury:*

- Full-body check including skin, face, chest, abdomen, muscles, nerves, and psychological condition.
- Diagnostic tests may be needed for internal damage.
- Record victim's story, injury timing, medical history, abuse setting. Torture methods are:
- Beating the soles of feet
- Amputation
- Suspension (hanging by limbs)
- Positional torture

*7. Firearm injury:*

- Caused by any weapon that fires projectiles using explosive force (e.g., gun, pistol, shotgun).
- Material used in the explosion (bullet, pellets, powder). Classification of firearms:

A. Barrel type:

- Smooth bore firearm (e.g., shotgun)
- Rifled firearm
- Country-made firearm
- Air gun
- Paradox gun

B. Muzzle velocity:

- Low velocity (up to 1200 ft/s) – e.g., revolver, pistol
- Medium velocity (1200–2500 ft/s)
- High velocity (>3000 ft/s) – e.g., machine gun.

***Structure of a Firearm***

- Barrel: Hollow steel tube or cylinder that directs the bullet.
- Bore: Inside diameter of the barrel.
- Stock or Grip: Handle of the firearm.

**Cartridge:**

***1. Detonator:***

- Ignites the gunpowder.
- Purpose: To create the initial spark to fire the bullet.

***2. Propellant:***

- Placed next to the primer.
- Primer ignition causes the gunpowder to burn, creating hot gases.
- Gases build pressure to eject the bullet or pellets from the firearm.
- Types of Gunpowder: Black Powder, semi-smokeless powder, smokeless powder.

***Bullet Structure:***

- Bullets are usually conical in shape.
- Parts:

1. Base – Flat part inside the cartridge.
2. Body – Main cylindrical portion.
3. Nose – Tip of the bullet.

***Types of Bullet Nose Shapes:***

- Round nose
- Square nose

- Pencil point nose
- Flat point
- Long round nose
- Rifled firearms cause two wounds: Entry wound (where bullet enters) and Exit wound (where bullet leaves).

Table 21.1

| Entry wound | Exit wound |
|---|---|
| Small in size | Outward split edges |
| On skull: outer surface cut and chipped inward | Bevelled and everted edges |
| Edges are inverted | Exerted edges |
| Abrasion collar is present | Abrasion collar is absent |
| Burning and blackening is seen | Usually not seen |
| Clothes turned in and carried into wound | Clothes may or may not be turned out |
| Entry track may appear bright pink | Track usually not pink |
| Lead ring seen in X-ray | Lead ring absent |

***Tests Used in Firearm Discharge***

1. Tests for detecting Nitrate:

- Dermal nitrate test or Paraffin test→ Checks for presence of nitrates on the hand (from gunshot residue).

2. Tests for detecting Heavy Metals:

- Harrison and Gilroy test: Detects antimony, barium, lead.
- Neutron activation analysis: Detects antimony and copper.
- Atomic absorption spectroscopy: Detects antimony, barium, copper.

**Explosion injury:**

- An explosion injury occurs due to sudden release of energy, causing a blast wave, and movement of objects or heat.
- Types of explosion injury:

1. Primary – From shock waves affecting hollow organs (ears, lungs, intestines, etc.).
2. Secondary – From flying debris or shrapnel.
3. Tertiary – From blast wind throwing the victim into other objects.
4. Quaternary – From complications like asphyxia or respiratory failure.

***Motor vehicle injury:***

1. Two wheeler injury:

- Motorcyclist fracture: A hinge fracture at the base of the skull (divides into front and back).
- Ring fracture: A circular fracture around the foramen magnum of the skull.
- Bicycle spoke injury: Leg/foot gets caught in wheel spokes.
- Tailgating injury: A motorcyclist crashes into a car due to sudden stop.

2. Four wheeler injury:

- Sparrow foot marks: Small cuts from shattered windshield
- Hinge fracture
- Ladder tears
- Seatbelt syndrome: Injuries from seatbelt – may include internal organ damage
- Whiplash injury: Neck injury from sudden jerking (front and back motion)
- Steering wheel injury: Injury from hitting steering wheel during crash

**Pedestrian Injuries: Waddle's Triad – 3 types of injuries**

***1. Primary Impact Injuries:***

- Caused when a vehicle first hits the person.
- May leave imprint, abrasion, or patterned bruise

*2. Secondary Impact Injuries:*

- Caused by same vehicle during subsequent contact.
- Leads to head injury, laceration, and run-over injuries.
- Occurs on same side as primary impact.

*3. Secondary Injuries:*

- Caused by falling on ground or hitting a stationary object.
- Seen on opposite side of primary impact.
- Common Sites in Pedestrians: Legs (85%), Head, Arms, Pelvis, Chest or abdomen, Neck and spine.

**Regional injuries:**

***Head Injuries***

(A) Scalp Injuries:

- Scalp bruises are often swollen (oedematous)
- Best detected by touch (palpation) rather than shaving
- Can be mistaken for incised wounds due to thinness of scalp

Features:

- May show abrasions, lacerations, bruises
- Helps identify point of contact
- Bruises may move under the skin over time

(B) Skull Injuries:

- Skull is complex; hence, fractures vary based on impact and location.
- Mechanism of skull fractures includes:
- Direct blow to the head
- Fall from height
- Compression or crushing injury

***Types of Skull Fractures:***

1. Linear Fracture:

- Straight line fracture
- Commonly occurs in the temporal and parietal bones

2. Depressed Fracture:

- Bone is pushed inward
- Caused by heavy blunt object (e.g., hammer)

3. Comminuted Fracture:

- Bone broken into multiple pieces
- Seen in high impact trauma

4. Basilar Fracture:

- Involves base of the skull
- Signs: Raccoon eyes, Battle's sign, CSF leakage

5. Ring Fracture:

- Around foramen magnum
- Seen in falls from height or severe spinal injury

***Medico-Legal Importance of Head Injuries:***

- Helps determine nature of weapon used.
- Can establish cause and manner of death (accidental, homicidal, suicidal).
- Shows direction and force of impact.
- Timing of injury (age) may be inferred.
- Important for legal documentation and court evidence.

(C) Intracranial injury:

1. Intracranial Hemorrhage:

- Fractures of the skull vault (top of the head) may travel down to the base, meeting in the pituitary fossa — forming a hinge fracture.
- The bleeding pattern depends on the anatomy of blood vessels.
- Meningeal arteries are usually safe unless there are fractures crossing their path.

2.Extradural hemorrhage:

- Usually involves the middle meningeal artery.
- Presents as a "lucid interval" (consciousness for ~30 mins to 1 hr) followed by deterioration.

3.Subdural hemorrhage:

- From damage to communicating veins.
- Not always due to skull fractures.
- Recent subdural: Dark red, seen under microscope with Perl's stain.
- Chronic subdural: Seen in elderly or frequent fall patients due to brain shrinkage.

(D) Traumatic Subarachnoid Hemorrhage:

- Small hemorrhages from trauma or brain movement inside the skull.
- Large ones can occur due to neck trauma.
- Most are non-traumatic, caused by bursting of aneurysms (Circle of Willis).

(E) Brain Injury:

- Caused by skull fracture or internal bleeding due to trauma.
- Whole brain is affected, may lead to cerebral edema (swelling).
- Direct injuries: Skull fragments bruise or cut brain cortex.
- Penetrating injuries: Bullets/stabs can damage deep brain areas

(F) Neck Injuries:

Forensic importance:

1. Many vital structures are present in the neck.
2. It is vulnerable to injury.

- Post-mortem: Done via layer-by-layer dissection.
- Penetrating trauma (sharp weapons/bullets): Can cause damage to arteries, veins, airway, etc.

- Incised wounds: Carry more forensic value than blunt trauma.

(G) Spinal Injuries:
Common due to:
1. Major trauma.
2. Atlanto-occipital joint disruption (between head and neck).

(H) Thoracic Injuries (Chest)
- Inward injuries: Suspicious if arteries are injured.
- Outward injuries: May result in air escaping (pneumothorax).

(I) Abdominal Injuries:
- Blunt force injuries (especially from front/back pressure) may injure internal organs, such as:

1. Bruising or rupture of:
- Duodenum or jejunum
- Pancreas
- Liver

2. Disruption of:
- Omentum (fatty layer)
- Mesentery (connects intestines)

***Thermal injuries:***

Thermal injuries are caused by exposure to heat or chemicals. They are classified into: Explosive burns, Scalds, Chemical burns, Radiation burns, Electric burns.

***1. Burns (Simple Burns):***

- Simple burns occur from dry heat.
- Minimum burn temperature: ~44°C.
- Exposure of 5–6 seconds at this temperature can cause burns.
- At 65°C, burns happen in just 2 seconds.

- Full-thickness burns occur if temperature is above 70°C.

*Degree of Burns:*

- Burns are classified into six degrees (Dupuytren's classification), merged into three types:

***1. Epidermal Burns (1st & 2nd degree):***

- Affected skin becomes red (erythematous).
- Capillaries dilate; fluid leaks into tissue causing swelling.
- Painful but usually heals without scarring.

***2. Dermo-epidermal burns (3rd & 4th degree):***

- Full skin thickness is destroyed.
- Burned area appears shriveled and sunken.
- Painless due to nerve destruction.
- Coagulated tissue with red blisters.

***3. Deep burns (5th & 6th degree):***

- Severe damage to skin, subcutaneous tissue, muscles, and bones.
- No pain as nerves are destroyed.

*Burn index:*

- 0.5 point per 1% of 2nd-degree burns
- 1 point per 1% of 3rd-degree burns
- 45 points = ~50% mortality

*Extent of Burns:*

- Extent of surface area burned is crucial in prognosis:

***Adults – Rule of Nine (Wallace's formula):***

1. Head and neck – 9%
2. Each upper limb – 9%
3. Front of each lower limb – 9%

4. Back of each lower limb – 9%
5. Front of chest – 9%
6. Back of chest – 9%
7. Front of abdomen – 9%
8. Back of abdomen – 9%
9. Genitalia – 1%

Image 21.1 Wallace's rule of nine

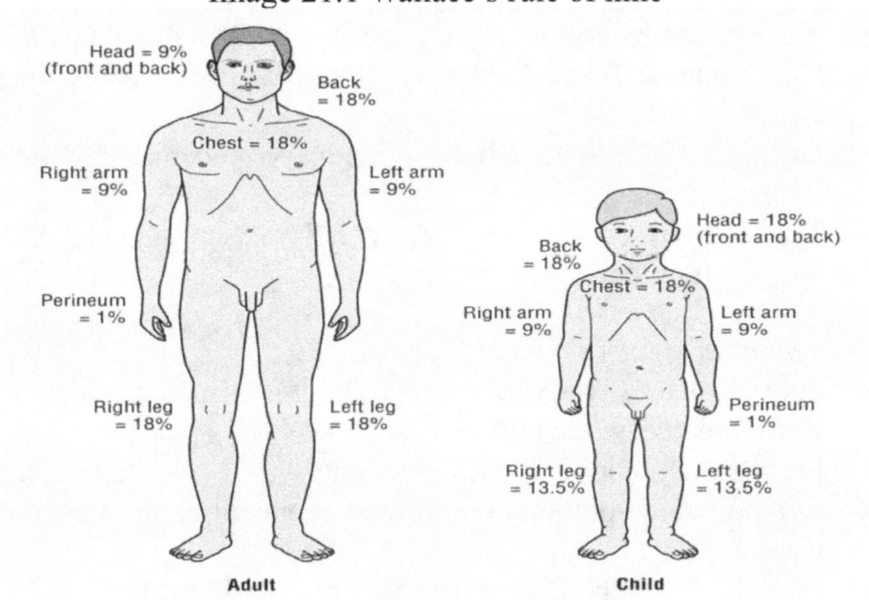


Table 21.2 Lung and browder chart

| | **1-4 years** | **5-9 years** | **10-14 years** |
|---|---|---|---|
| **Head and neck** | 19 | 15 | 13 |
| **Trunk front** | 16 | 16 | 16 |
| **Trunk back** | 16 | 16 | 16 |
| **Upper limbs** | 19 | 19 | 19 |
| **Lower limbs** | 30 | 34 | 35 |
| **Genitals** | 0 | 0 | 1 |

- Genitals: 0% up to 9 years; in children, head is the largest surface area.
- Palm surface: ~1% of total body surface (used to estimate burn size).

***Causes of death in burn:***

- Shock: Due to fluid and plasma loss.
- Infection: Burn wounds are prone to bacterial infections.
- Toxaemia: Absorption of toxic substances from burned tissue.
- Other causes: Renal failure, respiratory failure, multi-organ failure.
- Fat embolism, suffocation, pulmonary oedema, Cyanide intoxication.
- The delayed causes are: kidney failure, sepsis, gangrene, tetanus, liver damage.

***Post-mortem signs in burns:***

- Soot in airways (larynx, trachea, lungs) → indicates person was alive during the burn.
- Carboxyhemoglobin (>5%) gives cherry-red color to blood.
- Cyanide may be found in blood, depending on material burned.
- Pugilistic attitude: Due to heat-induced muscle stiffening.
- Looks like boxing or fencing posture.
- Caused by protein coagulation.

**Special Post-mortem finding:**

***Heat Ruptures (Heat Split Fissures)***

- Common on stretched areas like back of arm, joints
- Look like cuts but:

1. Nerves and vessels visible inside
2. No bleeding
3. Irregular edges
4. No signs of bruising

*Heat Hematoma:*

- Caused by heat; appears in head.
- Bilateral, soft, dark, shaped like a sickle.
- Looks like chocolate-colored jelly.
- No external injury

*Ante-Mortem Burn Signs:*

- Redness, swelling, inflammation
- Vital reaction present
- Clear line of demarcation
- Real blisters with albumin + chloride
- Fluid-filled blisters with hard yellow walls
- Enzyme reaction in skin
- Increased serotonin & histamine
- Curling ulcers may appear in duodenum after 1 week

- **Other Thermal Injuries:**

***1. Electric burns:***

- Also called Joule Burns.
- Caused when electric current passes through body, generating internal heat

Types of electric burns:

- Contact burns – from touching live wires
- Flash burns – due to electric arcs
- High voltage injuries – deep tissue damage
- Electric marks (Joule burns) – entry/exit points
- Burn marks may be found on clothes or shoes.
- Usually includes an entry wound and an exit wound:

*i) Entry Wound:*

- Thick, dry, grey-white, depressed area
- Non-bleeding, hard, cauliflower-like
- Looks like a crater or crocodile skin
- May show different colors:
- Green: Brass electrode
- Black: Iron electrode
- Blue: Copper electrode
- Grey: Aluminium electrode

*ii) Exit Wound:*

- Lacerated and bleeding wound.
- Electrode metals may melt and deposit as metal pearls in the tissue..
- Calcium phosphate from bones may also melt (seen as wax dripping).
- Muscles may show Zenker's degeneration.

***2. Lightening burns:***

- Lightning burns are caused by discharge of electric current between a negatively charged cloud and a positively charged object on earth.

*Mechanism of Lightning Injury:*

- Direct effect of high voltage
- Heat (superheated air causes burns)
- Blast wave from air expansion
- Sledge hammer blow: Body thrown due to compressed air before current hits.

*Characteristic Finding:*

- Lichtenberg Figures (also called arborescent burns).
- Appear as branched, tree-like red patterns on skin (especially shoulders and flanks).

- Do not follow blood vessels.

***Dowry deaths:***

- When a newly married women are tortured or killed by husband or relatives due to dowry demands.

**Law Related to Dowry Death:**

***A) Section 304B IPC:***

- If a woman dies within 7 years of marriage under suspicious circumstances (e.g. burns, injury), and she was being harassed for dowry → husband or in-laws can be punished.
- Minimum 10 years imprisonment which can be extended.

***B) Section 498A IPC:***

- Punishes cruelty to a married woman by husband or his relatives.
- Cruelty = physical or mental harm, or harassment for dowry.
- Punishment: Up to 3 years imprisonment and fine.

**Dowry Death Investigation – Evidence Laws:**

***Section 113A IEA:***

- Presumption of abetment of suicide by husband/relatives in cases of cruelty

***Section 113B IEA:***

- Presumption of dowry death if woman dies under suspicious circumstances within 7 years of marriage and faced dowry-related cruelty

***Section 174(3) CrPC:***

- Autopsy (postmortem) is mandatory if a woman:
- Dies an unnatural death within 7 years of marriage, or
- Is below 30 years of age

***Section 176 CrPC:***

- Allows a magistrate to conduct inquest/investigation.

**Dowry prohibition act: (1961)**

- Taking or giving dowry is a punishable offence.
- Minimum 5 years imprisonment.
- Fine: At least Rs.15,000 or the value of the dowry, whichever is greater.

**Multiple Choice Questions**

**1. Which of the following is not a blunt wound?**

A. Laceration B. Contusion C. Stab wound D. Abrasion

**2. The shape or pattern of the object causing the injury is imprinted on the skin is**

A. Linear B. Graze C. Pattern D. Imprint

**3. Which of the following is not a bullet nose shape?**

A. Flat B. Linear C. Triangle D. Square

***4. Percentage of each upper limb is Wallace's rule?***

A. 9% B. 18% C. 30% D. 20%

**5. There is no pain in which degree of burn?**

A. 1st B. 2nd C. 4th D. 5th

**Answer key for MCQs:**

| | |
|---|---|
| 1 | C |
| 2 | D |
| 3 | C |
| 4 | A |
| 5 | D |

# Ch. 22
# Pregnancy, Delivery and Abortion

**Pregnancy:**

- A physiological state in females where conception occurs and the fetus develops in womb until birth.

**Medico-legal importance:**

***A) Civil cases:***

**1. Nullity of marriage:**

- A women is pregnant by other man before her marriage and conceals this fact then marriage can be declared null.

**2. Divorce:**

- If a woman becomes pregnant by another man before marriage and consummates marriage with her husband within a reasonable period, a decree of divorce may be granted.

**3. Breach of promise of marriage:**

- Pregnancy can be grounds for legal action.

**4. Alimony:**

- Pregnant women are entitled for higher maintenance allowances in divorce cases.

**5. Inheritance of property:**

- The unborn child has inheritance rights.

**6. Blackmailing:**

- Pregnancy can be used as a tool for blackmailing.

**7. Defamation:**

- Allegations related to pregnancy can result in defamation cases.

**8. Compensation:**

- If a pregnant women dies due to other's negligence, higher compensation is awarded.

**9. Plea to avoid court:**

- Pregnancy can be cited as a plea to avoid attending court.

***B) Criminal cases***

1. **Rape cases:** Pregnancy serves as a proof of sexual intercourse in rape cases.
2. **Suicide:** Pregnancy can be a cause of suicide in un-married woman.
3. **Murder motive:** Pregnancy can be the motive of murder if it results from illicit relations.
4. **Illicit sexual intercourse:** Pregnancy indicates such relations.
5. **Husband's suspicion:** A husband may kill his wife if he suspects infidelity.
6. **Execution of death sentence:** Under section 416 of CrPC, if a pregnant women is sentenced to death, the sentence is postponed or commuted to life imprisonment.

**Delivery:**

- The process of expelling the viable fetus from the womb at term.

**Medico-legal importance:**

***A) Civil cases:***

1. Pre-term or suspicious child birth
2. Affiliation and adaptation
3. Contested paternity

4. Child legitimacy
5. Nullity of marriage
6. Divorce
7. Inheritance of property
8. Higher alimony in divorce
9. Higher compensation in death of pregnant woman

***B) Criminal cases:***

1. Abortion
2. Infanticide
3. Concealment of birth
4. Blackmail
5. Judicial death sentence delay
6. Delivery as rape evidence
7. Homicide and suicide

**Impotence:**

- The persistent inability to develop or maintain a penile erection sufficient for intercourse.

*Causes:*

- **Endocrine**: Testicular failure, hyper-prolactinemia
- **Penile disease**: Peyronie's disease, priapism, trauma
- **CNS**
- **Vascular disease**: Atherosclerosis, stenosis of arteries
- **Drugs**: H2 blockers, beta blockers
- **Congenital**: Klinefelter syndrome
- **Chronic disease**: Diabetes, neuropathy
- **Psychological**: Anxiety, fear, guilt

*Medico-legal cases:*

- Impotence may be used as a defense in rape or unnatural sexual offence.

*A) Civil cases:*

- **Nullity of marriage**: Wife may seek divorce on grounds of impotence.
- **Disputed paternity**: A man may deny paternity citing impotence.
- **Compensation**: Compensation can be claimed for injury causing impotence.

*B) Criminal cases:*

- **Plea in rape cases**: Impotence may be used as a defense
- **Adultery defense**: May be stated as a plea

**Types:** Temporary, Permanent

**Sterility:**

- It is the inability of a person to procreate.
- In males, it is the inability to fertilize the ovum while in females it is the inability to conceive.

*Types of female infertility:*

- **Relative**: Diminished capacity to recreate which can be treated.
- **Absolute**: Complete incapability to conceive which is untreatable.

***Based on state:***

- **Physiological**: Occurs at extreme ages.
  Eg: a child cannot procreate before puberty.
- **Pathological**: Caused by a disease or medical condition preventing procreation.

***Causes:***

***A) In males:***

- Extreme age

- Malformations: Hypospadias, epispadias
- Diseases: Azoospermia, oligospermia, orchitis
- Exposure to X-rays

***B) In females:***

- Extreme age
- Malformation: absence of ovum
- Diseases: Tuberculosis, endometriosis, PCOD, gonorrhea

**Medico-legal importance:**

- **Disputed paternity**: A man may claim he is sterile to deny fatherhood.
- **Compensation**: For loss of reproductive ability due to injury or occupation.
- **Adoption**: Sterility may be a plea in abortion cases.
- **Absolute sterility** in man may be a plea for artificial insemination.

**Sterilization:**

- It is a procedure to make the person infertile without affecting sexual potency.

***Types:***

1) **Voluntary**: With consent for contraception

2) **Compulsory**: Ordered by the government

***Methods:***

- **Male**: Vasectomy
- **Female**: Tubectomy

***Medico-legal importance:***

- Doctor liability if sterilization fails causing unwanted pregnancy.
- Adultery if vasectomy fails in males

- Disputed paternity
- Legitimacy of child
- Divorce

- ***Abortion:***

It is the expulsion of embryo or fetus before it can survive outside the uterus.

***Types:***

1. **Natural**: It is spontaneous or accidental, occurring without external intervention.
2. **Artificial**: Induced through artificial method.
    - Legal: Under the Medical Termination of Pregnancy act
    - Criminal: Illegal abortions

***Criminal abortion:***

- Governed by sections 312-316 IPC.
- Common in widows prevented from re-marrying due to social customs.
- Unmarried girls who become pregnant.

**Methods of criminal abortion:**

***1. Drugs:***

- Ecbolics: Ergot, quinine
- Emmenagogues: Synthetic estrogen, oil of savin, borax, apiol.

***2. Abortion stick:***

- Thin wooden or bamboo stick or irritant plant twigs
- Calotropis (madar)
- Nerium odonrum
- Plumbago zeylanica
- Plumbago rosea

***Infanticide:***

Killing a child after birth within 1 year of delivery.

***Medico-legal aspects:***

- Considered murder under section 302 of IPC.
- Every child is presumed born alive. In infanticide it is necessary to prove that child was born alive before being killed.
- Investigation is done to confirm if the child was alive at birth or still-born.

**Still-born:**

- A baby born after 28 weeks of pregnancy but showing no signs of life.
- The child may die in-utero just before delivery.
- A child that dies in the womb shows signs like:

  1. Rigor mortis
  2. Maceration:

- Aseptic autolysis in a dead fetus when retained in the uterus for 3-4 days.
- Skin slippage within 12 hours.
- Presence of gas in organs.
- Spalding's sign=overlapping skull bones.
- Foul smell

  3. Putefaction:

- If membranes rupture, air enters causing decomposition instead of maceration.
- Body becomes bloated, greenish and foul smelling.

  4. Mummification:

- Occurs when there is no air or fluid and poor blood supply.
- Body becomes thin, shriveled, dark brown and smells like rotten cheese.

***Live birth:***

- A child that shows any signs of life when born even when not fully expelled from mother.
- Even minimal signs like breathing, crying, heart pulsations or muscle movements indicate life.

**Virginity:**

- A virgin is a woman who has never had sexual intercourse.
- Defloration means loss of virginity.

***Signs of virginity:***

1. Labia majora: Thick, rounded, firm, fleshy, elastic and closely opposed.
2. Labia minora: Small, thick, pink, lying inside labia majora.
3. Clitoris: Small
4. Vestibule: Narrow
5. Vagina: Small, reddish, narrow with rugose walls.
6. Hymen: Intact
7. Fourchette and posterior commissure: Intact
8. Fossa navicularis: Normal

**Battered baby syndrome:**

- Also known as Caffey's syndrome, child abuse syndrome or non-accidental injury of child.
- Repeated abuse of child by parents or guardians.
- Usually affects children under 2 years.
- Slightly more common in male children.
- Evidence of neglect.
- Disproportionate soft tissue injuries with inconsistent history.
- Injuries at different times.
- History from caregivers doesn't match clinical finding.
- Multiple admissions to hospital.
- Often seen in broken families, low socio-economic status, children from unwanted pregnancies or illegitimate relations.

***Medico-legal importance:***

- In India, battered baby syndrome is low.
- If a child dies after live birth, the parents may face homicide charges.

**Hymen:**

- A thin mucous membrane at the vaginal opening with a small opening.
- Usually shaped annular or semilunar with broader part posteriorly.
- May be imperforate, cribriform, septate.
- Usually tears during first intercourse
    a. Postero-laterally at 4,5,7,8 o'clock position
    b. Sometimes posteriorly at 6 o'clock.
- In children, hymen is deep seated.
- Ulcerations, salaphite or constant itching may also cause the hymen to rupture.
- Hymen may also rupture due to local injuries, trauma, gynec procedures, masturbation with large objects, use of tampons.
- Activities like cycling, running, jumping, horse-riding don't rupture hymen.
- **Glaister keene rods** may help degree and timing of hymen rupture.

**Artificial insemination:**

- A procedure of transfer of semen into reproductive system of a woman without sexual intercourse.
- Types:
    a. Artificial insemination husband (AIH): Husband's semen is used.
    b. Artificial insemination donor (AID): Donor's semen is used.
- Indications:

*A) AIH:*

- Husband is impotent but fertile.
- Husband can't deposit semen due to malformations or hypospadias.

**B) AID:**

- Husband is sterile.
- Husband carries heredity genetic disorder.
- Couple has Rh-incompatibility.
- Woman is iso-immunized and prior pregnancies have failed.
- Husband has severe oligospermia and denies advanced ART like Intracytoplasmic Sperm Injection (ICSI).

***Medico-legal importance:***

- Legitimacy of child
- Adultery
- Nullity of marriage and divorce
- Inces

**Legitimacy of child:**

- A child is legitimate if

a) Born during valid marriage between parents.

b) Born within 280 days after divorce provided the mother remains unmarried.

***Important terms:***

- **Superfecundation**: Two ova fertilized during the same menstrual cycle by different fathers.
- **Superfetation**: Another ovum fertilized in a later cycle during pregnancy.
- May lead to Twins with different fathers, two children born with different maturity stages, delivery of 2 babies within 1-3 months apart.

c) Suppositious child:

- A child fraudulently claimed by a woman to her own without actually delivering it.

d) Posthumous child:

- Child born after death of his biological father.

**Medical Termination of Pregnancy (MTP):**

- Legalized abortion in India for cases where:
- There is a risk to woman's health.
- Result of contraception failure in a married woman.
- Pregnancy due to rape.
- The fetus is likely to be born with physical or mental defects.

***MTP Amendment Act 2020:***

- These are the expanded conditions of abortion for enhancing women's reproductive rights.
- Upto 20 weeks: Abortion on advice of 1 doctor.
- 20-24 weeks: Allowed on advice of 2 doctors in specific cases.
- After 24 weeks: Permitted if serious fetal abnormalities are confirmed by a state medical board.

**Grounds for Abortion under MTP Act:**

1. **Medical**: Mother's life is in danger and can cause severe health injuries.
2. **Humanitarian**: Rape causes pregnancy in minor or major girls and in mentally unstable patients.
3. **Eugenic**: Child being handicapped due to severe mental and physical inabilities.
4. **Socio-economic**: There is risk to mother's health due to lack of nutrition or other reasons.
5. **Failure of contraception devices**: The mental health of mother is seriously affected if there occurs pregnancy due to failure of any contraception devices. This is the unique feature

of law and allows abortion on special request.

**Recommendations:**

***A) Person who can perform abortion:***

- Only the registered medical practitioner in Obstetrics and gynecology having assisted at least 25 MTP.

***B) Where can abortion be done:***

- Hospital approved and maintained by government, Private hospitals having license from the Chief Medical Officer of district.
- Abortion is to be performed secretly and reported in a written form to the director of state.
- Upto 24 weeks termination allowed only when opinions of 2 doctors is taken along with the written consent of woman.
- In minors and lunatics, the written consent of a guardian is necessary.

**Pre-Conception and Pre-Natal Diagnostic Technique:**

- Sex ratio indicates the number of women per 1000 men in a population.
- Child sex ratio is number of boys to girls in age 0-6 years.
- A balanced sex ratio shows good social health.
- In developed societies, women generally out-number men.
- A low sex ratio shows social imbalance.
- The misuse of technology for sex determination has led to declining sex ratio.
- This creates barriers to sustainable social development.

***PCPNDT Act:***

- Enacted in 1994 and amended in 2003.
- The main aim is to prevent the misuse of diagnostic tools for sex selection and female foeticide.

***Purpose of the act:***

- To prohibit and regulate the use of diagnostic techniques for determining the sex of the fetus before or after conception.
- Prevent the sex-selective elimination of fetus.
- Establish institutional mechanisms to monitor diagnostic techniques.

***Provisions:***

- Ban on pre-natal sex determination.
- Provision of punishments and penalties for any violations.

***Objectives:***

- Ban sex-selection techniques before or after conception.
- Prevent misuse of pre-natal diagnostics techniques for sex-selective abortion.

***Salient features:***

- The offences under the act are:
    - Conduction of pre-natal sex determination using unregistered equipment or in unregistered centers.
    - Involvement in sex selection of a men or women.
    - Conducting PNDT tests for the purposes not allowed by the government.

**Main provisions of the act:**

***1. Prohibition of sex selection:***

- Bans the sex selection before or after the conception.

***2. Regulation of pre-natal diagnostic techniques:***

- Genetic abnormalities
- Metabolic disorders
- Chromosomal abnormalities
- Certain congenital mar
- Malformations

- Haemoglobinopathies
- Sex linked disorders

***3. Ban on sex determination tests:***

- No laboratory, clinic or center can conduct anytest, screening including USG to detect the sex.

***4. Confidentiality:***

- The sex of the fetus may not be disclosed to pregnant woman or anyone else by means of words or signs.

***5. Advertisement prohibited:***

- Advertising pre-natal or pre-conception sex determination by any means like notice, circular, label, hoarding, signs, light or sound is prohibited.
- The violation of any above rules can lead to
    - a) Imprisonment up to 3 years and
    - b) Fine up to Rs. 10,000

**Multiple Choice Questions**

**1. Which of the following can be a cause of impotence?**

A. Endocrine B. Trauma C. Mental D. All above

**2. Inability to fertilize the ovum is called as**

A. Virgin B. Sterility C. Abortion D. Impotence

**3. Criminal abortion comes under which section of IPC**

A. 310 B. 320 C. 316 D. 331

**4. Infanticide refers to killing of a child within how many years of delivery?**

A. 1 B. 3 C. 5 D. 7

**5. What is the meaning of defloration?**

A. Virginity B. Impotence
C. Loss of virginity D. Abortion

**6. Two ova released in the same cycle get fertilized is**

A. Superfecundation B. Superfetation
C. Suppositious D. None

**7. MTP act was revised in which year?**

A. 1919 B. 1975 C. 2003 D. 2019

**8. The battered baby syndrome is usually seen under what age?**

A. 2 B. 3 C. 4 D. 5

**9. The method of sterilization used in males is**

A. Tubectomy B. Vasectomy C. Laparoscopy D. None

**10. What lies under labia majora, is thin and pink?**

A. Clitoris B. Hymen C. Vestibule D. Labia minora

**Answer key for MCQs:**

| | |
|---|---|
| 1 | D |
| 2 | B |
| 3 | C |
| 4 | A |
| 5 | C |

| | |
|---|---|
| 6 | A |
| 7 | B |
| 8 | A |
| 9 | B |
| 10 | D |

# Ch. 23
# Sexual Offences

| Natural sexual offence | Unnatural sexual offence | Sexual perversions |
|---|---|---|
| Involves the use of sex organs in a natural way.<br>Eg: Rape, Adultery | Involves the use of sex organs against the order of nature.<br>Eg: Sodomy, Buccal coitus | Intended for sexual gratification with no sexual intercourse involved. |

### 23.1 Rape:

Rape is committed when sexual intercourse occurs under the following condition under section 375 IPC:

1. Without her consent and against the will
2. With her consent but
    a. She is less than 16 years of age
    b. Is intoxicated or has unsound mind
    c. Forced consent or injury to her near ones
    d. Consent obtained by impersonatio

**• Medico-legal aspect of rape:**

**1. Statutory rape:** Sexual intercourse with a woman who is below the legal age of consent even if she agrees is considered as rape.

**2. Consent age:**

- A girl below 16 if not wife, cannot give legal consent.
- A wife below 15 cannot give a legal consent.
- In India, a girl 16 or above can give the legal consent for

sexual intercourse.

**3. Marital exception:**

- Sexual intercourse by a man with his wife (above 15 years) is not a rape even if done against her consent.

**4. No minimum age for offender:**

- There is defined law below which a boy is incapable of rape.

**• Types of rape:**

***1. Custodial rape:***

- Committed by persons in authority when the woman is under their custody.
- Eg: Police officers, hospital staff.

***2. Gang rape:***

- When a woman is raped by a group of persons, all are deemed guilty if they act with a common intention.

***3. Date rape:***

- Sexual intercourse with a woman who is intoxicated unknowingly using sedative drugs during a social event like a date or party.
- Eg: Ketamine, GHB.

**• Examination in case of rape:**

**1. Examination of the victim:**

***A) Consent required:***

- Written informed consent is necessary before examining the victim.
- If the victim is above 12 years her consent is needed.
- If victim is below 12 years or un-sound, consent of a guardian or parent is needed.
- Female victims should be examined in the presence of a RMP

as per Section 53(2) of CrPC.

***B) Medical findings suggestive of rape:***

*i. Signs of struggle:*

- Tears, blood stains, semen or mud on clothes.
- Injuries like abrasions, bite marks, nail scratches om genitals.

*ii. Semen:*

- Presence of semen in vagina confirms sexual intercourse.

*iii. Spermatozoa:*

- Presence of spermatozoa is further important evidence of sexual intercourse.

***C) Lord's principle of exchange:***

- When two bodies come in contact there is exchange of materials.
- It can be cloth fibres, hairs, blood, saliva, semen, smegma from accused be found on victim & vice versa.

***D) Presence of smegma bacilli:***

- The presence of smegma is suggestive of sexual intercourse.

**2. Examination of the accused:**

***A) The accused can be examined without any consent under section 53(A) CrPC.***

***B) Findings suggestive of intercourse:***

iv. Torn frenulum:

- Indicates recent sexual intercourse.

*v. Smegma under prepuce:*

- Presence of smegma under foreskin is inconsistent with recent intercourse since it rubs off during intercourse and may be found under vagina.

- Smegma takes 24 hours to reform.
- If smegma is absent and no bath taken then it suggests intercourse.

*vi. Vaginal cells:*

- The vaginal cells present on penis are detected by Lugol's iodine test.

**• Laws related to rape:**

**1. IPC section 375:** Defines rape

**2. IPC section 376:** Specifies punishments for rape

  - 7 years of life imprisonment + fine (except if victim is his wife and not under 12 years).
  - If the raped woman is his wife (not under 12 years) then punishment can be 2 years imprisonment with or without fine.

**• Other unnatural sexual offences:**

- **Bestiality:** Sexual relation of a human with lower animals.
- **Tribadism:** A form of non-penetrative sexual activity between women where one woman rubs her genitals against her partner's.
- **Buccal coitus:** Refers to oral intercourse. Specifically inserting penis in mouth.

## 23.2 Sexual perversions:

***a. Sadism:***

- Sexual gratification through physical cruelty or pain on partner.
- Commonly includes biting, beating, whipping.

***b. Lust murder:***

- In extreme sadism, murder becomes a stimulus for sexual

arousal.

- It leads to erection, ejaculation, orgasm.

*c. Necrophagia:*

- Extreme sadism where a person mutilates a body and then sucks or licks wounds, bites the skin, drinks blood.

*d. Masochism:*

- Sexual pleasure is obtained by inflicting pain on one-self from their partner.
- They enjoy beating, enslaving or domination.

*e. Necrophilia:*

- Desire to eat dead bodies.

*f. Fetishism:*

- Sexual arousal by non-living objects or body pats.
- Eg: Undergarments, brassieres, petticoats, stockings.

*g. Transvestism:*

- A condition where a person gains satisfaction by dressing and behaving like opposite sex.
- Common in males having desire to behave like females.
- Often linked to sadomasochism.
- No hormonal or genital abnormality is involved.

*h. Masturbation:*

- Self stimulation to achieve sexual arousal.
- In males: done by moving penis against an object.
- In females: Gentle rubbing or pressure on clitoris or labis majora by fingers.
- It is an offence when done in public.

*i. Exhibitionism:*

- Intentional exposure of genitalia in public places for sexual pleasure.
- May or may not involve masturbation.
- Punishment: 3 months imprisonment + fine.

*j. Voyeurism:*

- Also known as Scoptophilia or peeping tom.
- Generally sexual pleasure is obtained by observing others in intimate situation without their consent.

*k. Frotteurism:*

- Sexual satisfaction by rubbing against people in crowd.
- Common in public places.
- People with perversion may have premature ejaculation or impotence when attempt made of sexual intercourse.

*l. Undinism:*

- Sexual pleasure felt by observing someone urinate regardless of their sex.

*m. Indecent assault:*

- Any act committed on female with intent or knowledge to outrage her modesty.
- Acts may include kissing, pressing breasts, exposing genitalis or thighs, inserting fingers in vagina, playing with vulva.
- These acts are considered as criminal offences.
- Can be punished under section 354 IPC upto 2 years imprisonment and/or fine.

***Paraphilias:***

- Refers to a condition where a person experiences intense sexual arousal or gratification through atypical objects or situations.

- Involves unusual fantasies, urges and behaviors.
- Focuses on non-human objects, humiliation and non-consenting individuals.
- Considered as a psychiatric disorder when involves harm to others.

**Multiple Choice Questions:**

**1. Sexual gratification through physical cruelty or pain on partner.**

A. Sadism B. Masochism C. Fetishism D. Masturbation

**2. What is also known as peeping tom?**

A. Undinism B. Voyeurism C. Sadism D. Masochism

**3. Which IPC section describes punishment for rape?**

A. 375 B. 376 C. 377 D. 378

***4. Sodomy is a type of which sexual offence?***

A. Natural B. Unnatural C. Perversion D. None

**5. Smegma under perpuce takes how many hours to reform?**

A. 24 B. 48 C. 12 D. 36

**Answer key for MCQs:**

| | |
|---|---|
| 1 | A |
| 2 | B |
| 3 | B |
| 4 | B |
| 5 | A |

# Ch. 24
# Forensic psychiatry

## 24.1 Common symptoms associated with psychiatric disorders:

- Psychiatric disorders can vary a lot in how they appear, but there are several common symptoms that often show up across different conditions.

### *1. Changes in Mood:*

- Persistent sadness, emptiness, or hopelessness
- Irritability or excessive anger
- Extreme mood swings (e.g., feeling very high or very low)

### *2. Disturbances in Thinking:*

- Persistent negative thoughts
- Trouble concentrating or making decisions
- Racing thoughts or slowed thinking
- Suspiciousness or paranoia

### *3. Changes in Perception:*

- Hallucinations (seeing, hearing, or feeling things that aren't there)
- Distorted sense of reality
- Feeling detached from self or surroundings (depersonalization/ derealization)

### *4. Behavioural Changes:*

- Withdrawal from friends, family, and activities
- Decline in work or school performance

- Risky or impulsive behaviour
- Aggression or agitation

***5. Cognitive Symptoms:***
- Memory problems
- Difficulty planning or organizing
- Confusion

***6. Changes in Sleep and Appetite:***
- Insomnia or oversleeping
- Eating much more or less than usual
- Unexplained weight loss or gain

***7. Physical Complaints Without Clear Medical Cause:***
- Fatigue or low energy
- Headaches, stomach aches, or body pains

***8. Suicidal Thoughts or Self-Harm:***
- Talking about wanting to die
- Self-injury (cutting, burning, etc.)
- Making suicide plans or attempts

**Lucid interval:**

In psychiatry, a lucid interval means a temporary period during which a person with a psychiatric disorder appears mentally clear, rational, and free of obvious symptoms before the illness again becomes apparent.

It's different from the lucid interval term in neurology/forensic medicine (e.g., after a head injury in epidural hematoma). In psychiatry, it's about brief remissions or periods of clarity in the course of a mental illness.

***Examples in Psychiatric Disorders:***

*1. Mania / Bipolar Disorder:*

- Between manic and depressive episodes, a patient may have a symptom-free phase (euthymic period).

*2. Schizophrenia:*

- Some patients experience short periods where hallucinations, delusions, and disorganization lessen, and they seem "normal" before symptoms recur.

*3. Delirium:*

- The patient may have fluctuating consciousness: confusion interspersed with lucid moments.

*4. Dementia:*

- Occasionally, patients may have brief episodes of improved orientation and coherent conversation before cognitive decline again becomes evident.

## 24.2 Civil and criminal responsibility of mentally ill person:

***A. Civil responsibility:***

**1. Management of Property:**

- An insane person may lose the ability to manage property.
- The court may appoint someone to handle it for them.

**2. Contracts:**

- Contracts made by an insane person are generally invalid.
- Exception: If made during a lucid interval, they may be valid.

**3. Marriage:**

- A marriage is invalid if either party was insane at the time of the ceremony.

**4. Competency as a Witness:**

- An insane person cannot give evidence in court.
- Exception: Allowed during a lucid interval.

**5. Consent:**

- Consent given by an insane person is invalid.

**6. Civil Rights:**

- Certain rights, such as voting or holding a driving license, are lost due to insanity.

**7. Guardianship:**

- An insane person cannot be a legal guardian of a minor or adopt a child.

**8. Testamentary Capacity:**

- Refers to the ability to make a valid will.
- An insane person can make a valid will only during a lucid interval.
- A holograph will is one written in the testator's own handwriting.

***B. Criminal responsibility:***

- In law, criminal responsibility means liability for punishment for crimes committed.
- Presumption: Every person is considered sane and accountable for their actions unless proven otherwise.
- A person proven to be insane is not responsible for their actions if they lack: Free will, Intelligence, Understanding of their acts.

- **McNaughten Rule (Legal Test of Insanity):**
- Origin: Daniel McNaughten (1843), who suffered from paranoid schizophrenia and shot a man by mistake, believing

he was persecuted.

**Principle:**

- A person is not criminally responsible if, at the time of the crime, they were suffering from a defect of reason due to mental illness, and:

1. Did not know the nature and quality of the act, or

2. Did not know the act was wrong.

- In India, reflected in Section 84 of IPC:

"Nothing is an offence if done by a person who, at the time of doing it, by reason of unsoundness of mind, is incapable of knowing the nature of the act, or that what he is doing is either wrong or contrary to law."

Table 24.1

| Doctrine | Main principle |
|---|---|
| Delusions and criminal responsibility | If a crime is committed under delusion, person is judged as if the delusional facts were real. |
| Doctrine of partial responsibility | If the person has some mental weakness and is not fully sane, they are partial responsible. |
| Durham rule | The person is not responsible if the act is due to mental instability. |
| Current rule | A person is not responsible, if at the time of crime, they lacked the capacity to regulate their conduct according to the law due to mental disease. |
| American Law Institute test | A person is not responsible if they lack the capacity to appreciate the wrongfulness of their act or to conform to the law, due to mental illness. |
| Norwegian system | No defendant considered insane is held criminally responsible. Very broad protection for the mentally ill. |

## 24. 3 Mental health act:

- The Mental Healthcare Act, 2017 (India) is the law that governs the rights, care, and treatment of people with mental illness in India.
- It replaced the Mental Health Act, 1987 and came into force on 7 July 2018.
- Key Features of the Mental Healthcare Act, 2017

### *1. Rights of Persons with Mental Illness:*

- Right to Access Mental Healthcare
  - Everyone has the right to affordable, quality mental health services without discrimination.

- Right to Live with Dignity:
  - No discrimination based on gender, religion, caste, culture, or financial status.

- Right to Confidentiality:
  - Medical records and personal details must be kept private.

- Right to Make Advance Directives:
  - A person can write instructions on how they want to be treated (or not treated) in the event they develop a mental illness in the future.

### *2. Decriminalisation of Suicide:*

- Attempt to commit suicide is not a criminal offence if the person was under severe mental stress.
- The government must provide care, treatment, and rehabilitation instead of punishment.

***3. Advance Directive:***

- A legal document where a person states:
- Preferred treatment.
- Treatments they do not want
- Person(s) to be appointed as their nominated representative

***4. Nominated Representative:***

- A trusted person chosen by the patient to take decisions regarding their mental healthcare if the patient cannot decide for themselves.

***5. Admission & Treatment:***

- Voluntary Admission: When the person seeks treatment willingly.
- Supported Admission: When the person is unable to make decisions but needs treatment.
- No person can be admitted or treated without their consent, except under specific conditions in the Act.

***6. Mental Health Review Boards (MHRB):***

- Independent bodies set up in each state to:
- Protect patients' rights.
- Review admission and treatment decisions.
- Handle complaints from patients or families.

***7. Responsibilities of Government:***

- Provide mental health services in every district.
- Ensure availability of essential medicines.
- Integrate mental health into general healthcare.
- Promote public awareness and reduce stigma.

***8. Protection from Cruel Treatment:***

- Prohibits chaining, solitary confinement, or electroconvulsive therapy without anaesthesia.

- Types of Admission:
    1. **Independent Admission** – When a person voluntarily seeks help and has the capacity to make decisions.
    2. **Supported Admission** – When a person lacks capacity and is admitted on the request of a nominated representative, with review board oversight.
- Importance:
    - Shifts focus from custodial care to rights-based, patient-centered care.
    - Aligns with UN Convention on the Rights of Persons with Disabilities (CRPD).
    - Reduces stigma and promotes rehabilitation

**Multiple Choice Questions:**

***1. Hallucinations come under changes of?***

A. Mood B. Perception C. Behaviour D. Thinking

**2. The person is not responsible if the act is due to mental instability is doctrine of?**

A. Durham B. Current C. Norwegian D. ALI

**3. Mental Healthcare Act came into force in**

A. 2012 B. 2015 C. 2017 D. 2019

**4. Some patients experience short periods where hallucinations, delusions, and disorganization**

A. Depression B. Bipolar Disorder
C. Dementia D. Schizophrenia

**5. McNaughten Rule came into origin in?**

A. 1847 B. 1844 C. 1843 D. 1841

**Answer key for MCQs:**

| 1 | B |
|---|---|
| 2 | A |
| 3 | C |
| 4 | D |
| 5 | C |

# Ch. 25
# Forensic Science Laboratory

## 25.1 Hierarchy and major divisions of Forensic lab services:

### *1. Hierarchy of Forensic lab services:*

- A forensic lab generally follows a top-down structure for administration and technical work.

Table 25.1

| Level | Designation | Role |
|---|---|---|
| Top management | Director / Chief Forensic Scientist | Head of the laboratory, policy-making, coordination with law enforcement and judiciary. |
| Senior management | Deputy Director / Additional Director | Supervises multiple divisions, ensures quality control, manages large cases. |
| Division heads | Director / Senior Scientific Officer | Heads a specific forensic division (e.g., biology, chemistry). |
| Scientists | Scientific Officer / Senior Scientific Assistant | Performs expert analysis, prepares reports, court testimony. |
| Technical staff | Laboratory Assistant / Technician | Prepares samples, maintains equipment, assists scientists. |
| Support staff | Administrative Officers, Clerks, Drivers | Logistics, record keeping, communication, maintenance. |

**2. Major Divisions of Forensic Laboratory Services:**

- A full-fledged forensic science laboratory (FSL) usually has these specialized divisions:

Table 25.2

| **Divisions** | **Specializations** | **Example of analysis** |
|---|---|---|
| Biology & Serology | Biological fluids, tissues | Blood grouping, semen detection, saliva analysis, hair examination |
| DNA Fingerprinting | Genetic identification | Criminal identification, paternity testing |
| Chemistry / Toxicology | Drugs, poisons, chemicals | Alcohol estimation, poison detection, narcotics analysis |
| Physics / Ballistics | Firearms, ammunition, tool marks | Gunshot residue analysis, bullet comparison |
| Questioned Documents | Handwriting, forgery detection | Signature verification, counterfeit currency |
| Fingerprints | Latent print development and comparison | Identification from crime scene prints |
| Cyber Forensics | Digital evidence | Computer/mobile data recovery, hacking investigation |
| Explosives | Bomb/explosive material | Identification of explosives, post-blast residue |
| Voice & Audio Analysis | Audio forensics | Speaker identification, audio tampering detection |
| Forensic Medicine / Anthropology | Skeletal remains | Age estimation, identification of remains |

## 25.2 Newer techniques and recent advantages: Polygraphy, narcoanalysis, DNA profiling:

***Polygraphy:***

- Polygraphy (popularly called the Lie Detector Test) is a forensic technique used to measure physiological responses while a person answers questions, in order to detect possible deception.

***A. Principle:***

- The polygraph works on the idea that lying produces measurable physiological changes due to stress or anxiety.
- It records multiple body functions simultaneously:
- Respiration rate
- Blood pressure & heart rate
- Skin conductivity (Galvanic Skin Response – GSR)

***B. Components of a Polygraph Machine:***

- Pneumograph: Measures breathing rate
- Cardiograph : Measures blood pressure & pulse
- Galvanometer: Measures skin conductivity
- Data Recording System: Graphically records changes on moving paper or digitally.

***C. Procedure:***

- Pre-test Interview – Examiner explains procedure, establishes rapport, and formulates relevant & control questions.
- Baseline Recording – Measures normal physiological values during neutral questions.
- Questioning Phase – Asks a mix of:
- Relevant questions (related to the crime)
- Control questions (emotionally charged but unrelated)
- Neutral questions (simple factual)
- Post-test Analysis – Examiner compares physiological responses to different question types.
- Interpretation – Based on patterns, determines if deception is likely.

***D. Applications in Forensics:***

- Criminal investigations (theft, murder, sexual assault)
- Screening in sensitive jobs (defense, intelligence agencies)

- Verification of witness statements
- Security clearance investigations

### *E. Limitations:*

- Not 100% reliable – anxiety, fear, or medical conditions can mimic deception signals.
- Requires trained examiners for accurate interpretation.
- Can be manipulated by some individuals (countermeasures).
- Admissibility in court – In India, polygraph results are not directly admissible as evidence, unless conducted with the subject's consent and supported by other evidence (per Supreme Court ruling, 2010).

### *F. Legal Position in India:*

a. Supreme Court (2010): Narco-analysis, Brain mapping, and Polygraphy cannot be conducted without consent.
b. Must be done voluntarily, with legal safeguards and presence of a lawyer.
c. Findings can guide investigation but cannot replace primary evidence.

## Narco-analysis:

- Narco-analysis is a forensic investigative technique in which a subject is given certain drugs (most commonly sodium pentothal or sodium amytal) that depress the central nervous system, putting them into a hypnotic or sedated state.
- In this state, it is believed that the person's ability to lie is reduced, and they may reveal truthful information.

### *A. Principle:*

- At lower doses, barbiturates slow brain activity and reduce a person's inhibitions.
- The subject enters a twilight state between consciousness and unconsciousness.

- In this state, imagination and fabricated responses are suppressed, making it more likely that responses are truthful.
- However, the person is still suggestible and can be influenced by the examiner's questions.

***B. Drugs Used:***

- Sodium Pentothal: Commonest drug used; induces drowsiness and relaxation.
- Sodium Amytal: Alternative; similar effects.
- Scopolamine: Sometimes used historically, less common now.

***C. Procedure:***

- **Medical Examination** – To check if the subject is fit for the procedure.
- **Intravenous Administration** – Drug given in controlled doses.
- **Onset of Sedation** – Person becomes drowsy but still responds to questions.
- **Questioning** – Investigators ask relevant questions about the crime.
- **Recording** – Session is audio-video recorded for review.
- **Medical Supervision** – Conducted under strict monitoring to avoid overdose.

***D. Applications in Forensic Science:***

- To get leads in criminal investigations.
- Used in cases where the suspect is uncooperative.
- To corroborate or contradict other statements.
- Sometimes applied in terrorism, kidnapping, or complex murder cases.

***E. Limitations:***

- Not full proof - Drugged statements may still be false, confused, or mixed with fantasy.

- Risk of suggestibility - The examiner's wording can influence answers.
- Medical risks - Respiratory depression, allergic reactions, coma in sensitive individuals.
- Ethical concerns – Infringement of personal rights and mental privacy.

*F. Legal Position in India:*

- Supreme Court of India, 2010 (Selvi vs State of Karnataka):
- Narco-analysis cannot be conducted without the informed consent of the subject.
- Must have a lawyer present during consent.
- Results not admissible as evidence in court, but can be used for investigation and to discover fresh leads.
- Voluntary administration + court permission + medical safeguards required.

**DNA Profiling:**

- DNA profiling (also called DNA fingerprinting or genetic fingerprinting) is a scientific technique used to identify individuals based on their unique genetic makeup.
- Since every person (except identical twins) has a unique DNA sequence, this method is used in forensic science, paternity testing, criminal investigations, and identification of remains.

*A. Principle:*

- DNA profiling is based on analyzing certain regions of DNA that show high variability between individuals.
- These are usually Short Tandem Repeats (STRs) or Variable Number Tandem Repeats (VNTRs) — sequences where small DNA units are repeated several times, and the number of repeats varies from person to person.

### *B. Steps in DNA Profiling:*

#### *Step 1: Collection of Samples.*

Biological materials such as blood, hair roots, saliva, semen, skin cells, or tissue are collected.

#### *Step 2: Extraction of DNA*

DNA is isolated from the cells using chemical or enzymatic methods.

#### *Step 3: Amplification (PCR)*

The specific DNA regions (like STRs) are amplified using Polymerase Chain Reaction (PCR) to make millions of copies.

#### Step 4: DNA Fragment Separation

The amplified DNA fragments are separated by Gel Electrophoresis or Capillary Electrophoresis according to size.

#### Step 5: DNA Pattern Detection

The separated DNA fragments are visualized (using fluorescent or radioactive markers).

The pattern of bands or peaks is the person's DNA profile or DNA fingerprint.

#### Step 6: Comparison

DNA profiles from different samples (crime scene vs suspect, child vs parents, etc.) are compared.

### *C. Applications of DNA Profiling*

- **Forensic Science** Identify suspects or victims in criminal cases, rape, or murder investigations
- **Paternity / Maternity Testing** Establish biological relationships
- **Identification** Identify bodies in mass disasters or missing person cases

- **Medical Diagnosis** Detect genetic disorders or inherited diseases
- **Anthropology / Evolution** Study genetic diversity and ancestry
- **Wildlife Forensics** Identify species or prevent poaching and illegal trade

*D. Legal and Ethical Aspects:*

- In India, DNA profiling is used under the guidance of the DNA Technology (Use and Application) Regulation Bill, 2019 (yet to be fully enacted).
- Must maintain privacy and consent; misuse of genetic data is strictly prohibited.
- DNA evidence is admissible in court if collected and analyzed properly.

*E. Techniques Used in DNA Profiling:*

- **RFLP (Restriction Fragment Length Polymorphism)** Older method using restriction enzymes and hybridization; time-consuming
- PCR-based STR analysisCurrent standard method; rapid and highly sensitive
- Mitochondrial DNA analysis: Used when nuclear DNA is degraded (e.g., in old bones, hair)
- **Y-chromosome analysis:** Used to trace paternal lineage or identify male contributors

*F. Advantages:*

- Highly accurate (probability of two unrelated people having the same DNA profile is $<$ 1 in a billion)
- Requires very small biological samples
- Helps solve criminal cases and identify missing persons

**Multiple Choice Questions:**

**1. What is the designation of top management in forensic lab services?**

A. Director B. Clerk C. Technician D. Assistant

**2. What are the number of steps in DNA profiling?**

A. 1 B. 2 C. 9 D. 6

**3. Skin conductivity measured by which polygraph machine?**

A. Galvanometer B. Pneumograph

C. Cardiograph D. None

**Answer key for MCQs:**

| | |
|---|---|
| 1 | A |
| 2 | D |
| 3 | A |

# Ch. 26
# Laws, Acts, Rules and Regulations

## 26.1 Clinical establishment act:

***Introduction:***

- Enacted by the Government of India in 2010.
- Objective: To regulate and register all clinical establishments in India, ensuring minimum standards of facilities and services.
- Applies to both public and private sector establishments (except those run by the Armed Forces).
- The Act came into force initially in 4 states (Arunachal Pradesh, Himachal Pradesh, Mizoram, Sikkim) and all Union Territories, but other states can adopt it.

***Objectives:***

1. To provide mandatory registration of all clinical establishments.
2. To prescribe minimum standards for facilities and services.
3. To ensure transparency in charges and maintain proper records.
4. To promote ethical practices in healthcare delivery.
5. To enable standardization in medical care across India.

***Scope:***

- Applies to all clinical establishments including:
- Hospitals
- Nursing homes
- Maternity homes
- Clinics, dispensaries
- Labs and diagnostic centers

- Single-doctor clinics (except some traditional healers)

**Key provisions:**

***1. Registration:***

- All establishments must register with a District Registering Authority.
- A provisional certificate is issued first, followed by permanent registration after inspection.

***2. Standards***

- Must comply with prescribed minimum standards for:
- Infrastructure
- Human resources (qualified staff)
- Equipment
- Records and reporting

***3. National register:***

- A central register is maintained for all clinical establishments in India.

***4. Rates of charges:***

- Hospitals must display and provide details of rates charged to patients.

***5. Records:***

- Maintenance and reporting of medical records is mandatory.

***6. Penalties:***

- Non-registration or violation of rules can lead to fines and closure of the establishment.

**Authorities under the act:**

***1. National Council for Clinical Establishments:***

- Headed by DGHS (Director General of Health Services).

- Advises the central government on standards and guidelines.

*2. State council for Clinical establishment:*

- Advises state governments on implementation.

*3. District Registering Authority:*

- Headed by District Collector/District Magistrate.
- Maintains local register and supervises establishments.

*Exemptions:*

- Establishments under Armed Forces.
- Some traditional and alternative healers (when notified by state).

*Significance:*

- Ensures quality and accountability in healthcare.
- Protects patients from malpractice and overcharging.
- Promotes uniformity in healthcare services across India.

**Salient Features of Clinical Establishments Act, 2010**

*1. Mandatory Registration*

- All clinical establishments (public and private) must be registered.
- Covers hospitals, nursing homes, clinics, labs, imaging centers, AYUSH establishments, etc.
- Exemption: Armed Forces' establishments.

*2. Uniformity standards:*

- Prescribes minimum standards of facilities and services.
- Standards relate to infrastructure, manpower, equipment, and records.

*3. Two stage registration:*

- Provisional registration → given initially.

- Permanent registration → after inspection and compliance.

***4. National and state registers:***

- A National Register of clinical establishments is maintained.
- State and district authorities maintain local registers.
- Coverage of all system

***5. National and state counsels:***

- National Council for Clinical Establishments → frames policies, standards, guidelines.
- State Councils → implement and monitor at the state level.
- District Registering Authority → responsible for local supervision.

***6. Transparency in charges:***

- Establishments must display and provide rates of procedures and services to patients.

***7. Maintenance of records:***

- Compulsory maintenance and reporting of patient and service records in standard formats.

***8. Coverage of all systems of medicines:***

- Applicable to Allopathy, AYUSH (Ayurveda, Yoga, Unani, Siddha, Homeopathy), dentistry, etc.

***9. Penalties for non-compliance:***

- Fine for non-registration, violation of provisions, or non-adherence to standards.
- May lead to cancellation of registration or closure.

***10. Focus on patient rights:***

- Aims to prevent malpractices, ensure accountability, and improve patient confidence in healthcare.

**State AYUSH registration rules and regulations:**

Table 26.1

| Aspect | Details |
|---|---|
| **Established under** | State AYUSH acts: guided by ministry of AYUSH |
| **Administered in** | Allopathic and AYUSH |
| **Registration required** | Mandatory for practice; proof of recognized qualification needed. |
| **Registration details** | Mandatory unique ID, registry entry, certificate, periodic renewal. |
| **Ethics and conducts** | Governed by NCISM, board code of ethics, violations penalized |
| **Disciplinary action** | Boards can suspend or cancel registration, appeals allowed. |
| **Scopes restrictions** | Cannot practice modern medicine without approval. |
| **Record keeping** | Case records, informed consent, adherence to safety guidelines required. |
| **Medico-legal role** | May act as expert witness in legal matters. |
| **Safety registration** | Guidelines for handling herbs and practices. |

## 26.2 Medicare service persons and Medicare service institutions:

***Background:***

- Passed in several states of India around 2008–2010 in response to increasing violence against doctors and healthcare workers.
- Aim: To protect medical professionals and institutions from assaults, threats, and damage to property during discharge of duties.
- Adopted with minor variations by different states (e.g., Maharashtra, Andhra Pradesh, Karnataka, etc.).

***Objectives:***

1. To provide legal protection to healthcare workers (Medicare service persons).
2. To safeguard healthcare facilities and institutions.
3. To treat violence against medical personnel or hospitals as a cognizable and non-bailable offence.
4. To prevent damage to hospital property.

**Key definition:**

***1. Medicare Service Person – includes:***

- Registered doctors (allopathic, dental, AYUSH, etc.)
- Nurses, medical students, paramedical staff
- Other staff notified by state government.

***2. Service Institution – includes:***

- Hospitals, nursing homes, dispensaries, clinics
- Diagnostic centers, medical teaching institutions
- Any place where healthcare is provided.

**Salient features:**

***1. Violence defined:***

- Causing harm, injury, obstruction, or intimidation to healthcare workers on duty.
- Causing damage or loss to hospital property.

***2. Offence category:***

- Cognizable (police can take action without court order).
- Non-bailable (bail not granted as a matter of right).
- Non-compoundable (cannot be settled outside court).

***3. Punishment:***

- Imprisonment up to 3 years.
- Fine up to Rs.50,000 (varies slightly by state).

***4. Compensation:***

- Offenders are liable to compensate double the amount of damage caused to hospital property

***5. Special provisions:***

- Police required to take immediate cognizance of complaints.
- Fast-track trials encouraged.

**Significance:**

- First legislation in India specifically to protect medical professionals.
- Acts as a deterrent against assaults on doctors, nurses, and hospitals.
- Reinforces safety and dignity of healthcare service providers.

**26.3 Drugs and cosmetics Act:**

**Introduction:**

- Enacted: 1940 (came into force in 1945).
- Objective: To regulate the import, manufacture, distribution, and sale of drugs and cosmetics in India.
- Ensures that drugs and cosmetics are:
- Safe
- Effective
- Conform to prescribed quality standards.

***Objectives:***

1. To regulate manufacture and sale of drugs and cosmetics.
2. To ensure standards of quality, safety, and efficacy.
3. To prevent adulteration, spurious or substandard drugs.
4. To control misbranding and misleading advertisements.
5. To regulate the import of drugs and cosmetics into India.

***Scope:***

- Applies to Allopathy, AYUSH, biological and veterinary

drugs, cosmetics.

**Key provisions:**

***1. Regulatory Authorities***

- Central Drugs Standard Control Organization (CDSCO) – central authority.
- Drug Controller General of India (DCGI) – head of CDSCO, responsible for approval of new drugs, clinical trials, and regulation.
- State Drug Control Authorities – regulate manufacturing, sale, and distribution at state level.

***2. Drug Technical Advisory Board (DTAB)***

- Advises central/state governments on technical matters under the Act.

***3. Drug Consultative Committee (DCC)***

- Coordinates between central and state authorities for uniform implementation.

***4. Standards and Schedules:***

- Various Schedules under the Act specify requirements:
- Schedule G, H, H1, X → prescription-only drugs.
- Schedule M → good manufacturing practices (GMP).
- Schedule Y → clinical trial rules
- Schedule T → requirements for AYUSH medicines

***5. Licensing:***

- Mandatory license for manufacture, sale, and distribution.
- Import of drugs requires approval from central licensing authority.

***6. Labelling and packaging:***

- Clear mention of ingredients, strength, expiry, and batch

number.

- Warning labels for certain drugs.

***7. Penalties:***

- Manufacture or sale of spurious/adulterated drugs → imprisonment (up to life) + fine.
- Misbranding or sale without license → imprisonment + fine.

***Amendments:***

- 1964 → included Ayurvedic, Siddha, and Unani drugs.
- 1982 → strengthened quality control provisions.
- 2008 & 2013 → stricter penalties for spurious drugs.
- 2020 Rules → related to medical devices (classified as drugs under the Act).

***Significance:***

- Protects public health by ensuring access to safe and effective medicines.
- Prevents exploitation through spurious or substandard drugs.
- Provides a legal framework for drug regulation in India.

## 26.4 The Occupation safety, health, working condition code, 2020:

***Objective:***

To consolidate and amend the laws regulating the occupational safety, health and working conditions of persons employed in an establishment and related matters, ensuring workers' safety, health, and welfare.

***Laws subsumed:***

- The OSH Code, 2020 subsumes 13 existing labor laws, including:
- The Factories Act, 1948
- The Mines Act, 1952

- The Dock Workers (Safety, Health and Welfare) Act, 1986
- The Contract Labour (Regulation and Abolition) Act, 1970
- The Inter-State Migrant Workmen (Regulation of Employment and Conditions of Service) Act, 1979
- The Working Journalists and Other Newspaper Employees Act, 1955
- The Motor Transport Workers Act, 1961
- The Beedi and Cigar Workers Act, 1966
- The Cine-Workers and Cinema Theatre Workers Act, 1981
- The Building and Other Construction Workers Act, 1996
- The Plantation Labour Act, 1951
- The Sales Promotion Employees Act, 1976
- The Working Journalists (Fixation of Rates of Wages) Act, 1958

***Applicability:***

- Applies to establishments employing 10 or more workers, except for mines, docks, and plantations where it applies irrespective of the number.
- Covers all employees, including inter-state migrant workers, contract labourers, and workers in unorganized sectors.

**Key features:**

***1. Registration of Establishments:***

- Mandatory online registration for all establishments.
- A single registration in place of multiple under different laws.

***2. Duties of Employers***

- Ensuring a workplace free from hazards.
- Provision of free annual health check-ups.
- Providing appointment letters to all employees.
- Ensuring proper working hours and leave.

***3. Duties of Employees***

- Comply with safety and health requirements.
- Report unsafe conditions.

***4. Working Hours & Leave:***

- Daily working limit fixed at 8 hours.
- Overtime provisions with double wages.
- Night shifts regulated, especially for women.

***5. Special Provisions for Women Workers***

- Women allowed to work in all types of establishments, including night shifts, with consent and adequate safety measures.

***6. Contract & Inter-State Migrant Workers:***

- Contractors employing 50 or more workers must provide certain facilities.
- Inter-state migrant workers are entitled to journey allowance, displacement allowance, and benefits equal to local workers.

***7. Health, Safety & Welfare:***

- Mandatory safety standards for factories, mines, construction sites, and dock work.
- Welfare facilities like canteens, first-aid, crèches, and welfare officers in larger establishments.

***8. Inspector-cum-Facilitators***

- Inspectors now act as facilitators for compliance rather than just enforcing penalties.

***9. Penalties***

- Heavy penalties for non-compliance (up to Rs.3 lakh fine and imprisonment for repeated violations).

***Significance:***

- Simplifies compliance by merging 13 laws into one code.
- Brings uniformity in regulations across sectors.
- Expands coverage to a larger workforce, including migrants and unorganized workers.
- Balances employer obligations with employee rights.

## 26.5 Employees State Insurance Act, 1948

***Objective:***

- To provide social security and health insurance benefits to employees and their dependents in cases of sickness, maternity, disability, employment injury, or death.

***Applicability:***

- Extends to factories and establishments (factories, shops, hotels, cinemas, road transport, medical/educational institutions, etc.).
- Threshold: Establishments with 10 or more employees (in some states, threshold is 20).
- Wage ceiling: Employees earning up to Rs.21,000/month (Rs.25,000/month for persons with disability) are covered.
- Applies in notified areas only.

***Administration:***

- The scheme is managed by the Employees' State Insurance Corporation (ESIC), an autonomous body under the Ministry of Labour & Employment, Govt. of India.
- ESIC runs hospitals, dispensaries, and provides funds for benefits.

***Contribution:***

- Employer's share: 3.25% of wages.
- Employee's share: 0.75% of wages.
- Total: 4% of wages.

***Benefits under ESI act:***

- Medical Benefit – Complete medical care for insured person + family.
- Sickness Benefit – 70% of wages for 91 days in a year (with medical certificate).
- Extended Sickness Benefit – Up to 2 years for chronic diseases (e.g., TB, cancer).
- Maternity Benefit – Full wages for 26 weeks (extendable). Covers confinement, miscarriage, adoption.
- Disablement Benefit:
- Temporary: 90% wages during disablement period.
- Permanent: Monthly pension based on % loss of earning capacity.
- Dependents' Benefit – Pension to dependents if employee dies due to employment injury/disease.
- Funeral Expenses – Lump sum of Rs.15,000 to family.
- Other Benefits – Vocational rehab, confinement expenses, unemployment allowance (Rajiv Gandhi Shramik Kalyan Yojana).

***Significance:***

- First comprehensive social security law for industrial workers in India.
- Provides healthcare + income protection to workers and their families.
- Ensures employer accountability in case of occupational risks.

## 26.6 Rights of Persons with Disabilities Act, 2016

***Objective:***

- To give effect to the UN Convention on the Right.
- Persons with Disabilities (UNCRPD), ratified by India in 2007.
- To protect the rights of persons with disabilities and ensure their full participation, equality, and dignity in society.

*Key features:*

**(a) Types of Disabilities Recognized.**

- The Act increased the list from 7 (in 1995 Act) to 21 disabilities, including:
- Locomotor disability, visual impairment, hearing impairment, speech and language disability
- Intellectual disabilities (specific learning, autism spectrum disorder)
- Mental illness, chronic neurological conditions, multiple sclerosis, Parkinson's.
- Blood disorders (hemophilia, thalassemia, sickle cell disease)
- Multiple disabilities including deaf-blindness

**(b) Rights and Entitlements:**

***1. Equality & Non-Discrimination***

- No person with disability shall be discriminated against in any matter relating to education, employment, access to public places, etc.

***2. Education***

- Free education for children with disabilities between 6–18 years.
- Inclusive education in neighbourhood schools.

***3. Employment:***

- 4% reservation in government jobs for persons with benchmark disabilities ($\geq$40%).
- Private sector encouraged to employ persons with disabilities.

***4. Reservation in higher education:***

- 5% seats reserved for persons with benchmark disabilities.

***5. Social security and healthcare:***

- Provision of schemes, insurance, rehabilitation services, and barrier-free access to public buildings.

***6. Legal Capacity:***

- Equal recognition before the law, right to own property, control financial affairs, and access justice.

***7. Special provisions for women and children:***

- Protection from abuse, exploitation, and neglect.

**(c) Institutional mechanism:**

- Chief Commissioner for Persons with Disabilities (CCPD) at the national level.
- State Commissioners at the state level.
- District-level committees to monitor implementation.

**(d) Penalties:**

- Discrimination or violation of provisions may lead to fines and imprisonment.
- For atrocities against persons with disabilities: imprisonment of 6 months to 5 years plus fine.

***Significance:***

- Aligns Indian law with international standards (UNCRPD).
- Expands the scope of recognized disabilities.
- Provides affirmative action in education and jobs.
- Strengthens institutional framework for grievance redressal.

**Multiple Choice Questions**

**1. Clinical establishment act was Enacted by government in?**

A. 2010 B. 2011 C. 2012 D. 2013

**2. Persons with Disabilities (UNCRPD), ratified by India in**

A. 2007 B. 2008 C. 2009 D. 2010

**3. Drugs and cosmetics Act came into force in**

A. 1986 B. 1999 C. 1945 D. 2000

**4. Drugs and cosmetics Act Enacted in?**

A. 1943 B. 1944 C. 1940 D. 1938

**5. Maternity Benefit with full waged in employees state insurance Act is for how many week?**

A. 17 B. 26 C. 16 D. 34

**Answer key for MCQs:**

| | |
|---|---|
| 1 | A |
| 2 | A |
| 3 | C |
| 4 | C |
| 5 | B |

www.ingramcontent.com/pod-product-compliance
Lightning Source LLC
Chambersburg PA
CBHW062132160726
48282CB00027B/803